THE 28-DAY GOUT DIET PLAN

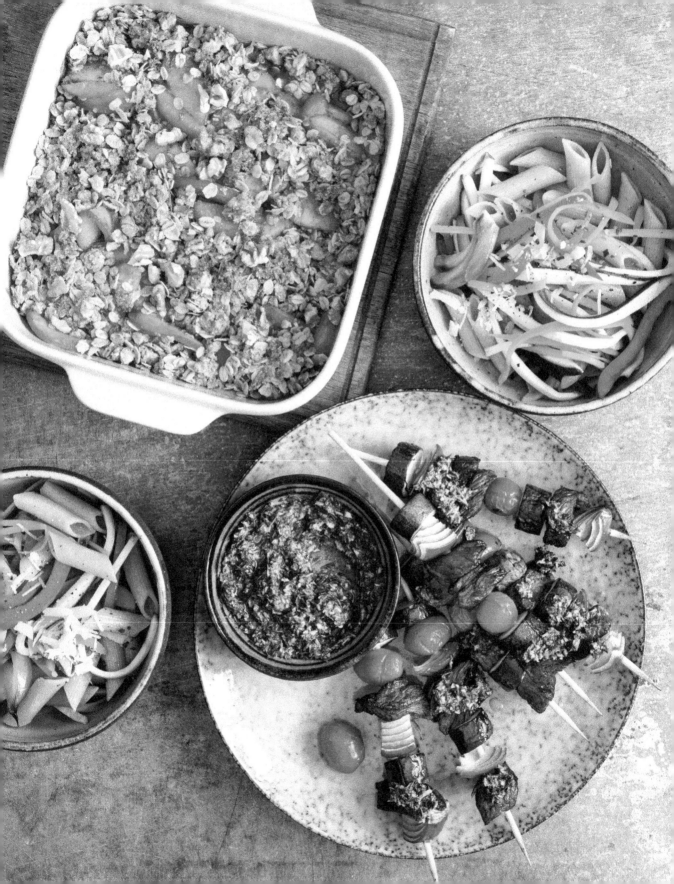

THE 28-DAY
GOUT DIET PLAN

The Optimal Nutrition Guide to Manage Gout

SOPHIA KAMVERIS, MS, RD, LDN

Foreword by Arun Mukherjee, MD, MRCP, FACP
Photography by Nadine Greeff

**ROCKRIDGE
PRESS**

For general information on our other products and services or to obtain technical support, please contact our Customer Care Department within the U.S. at (866) 744-2665, or outside the U.S. at (510) 253-0500.

Rockridge Press publishes its books in a variety of electronic and print formats. Some content that appears in print may not be available in electronic books, and vice versa.

Interior and Cover Designer: Liz Cosgrove
Photo Art Director: Sue Smith
Editor: Salwa Jabado
Production Editor: Andrew Yackira
Photography by Nadine Greeff, 2018.

ISBN: Print 978-1-64152-198-7
eBook 978-1-64152-199-4

For Pete and Marge, for always looking after their baby sister;
sweet Ginny, who inspires me;
and for my love, David, who never lets me fall.

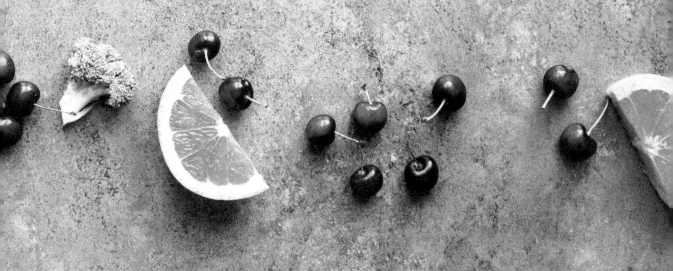

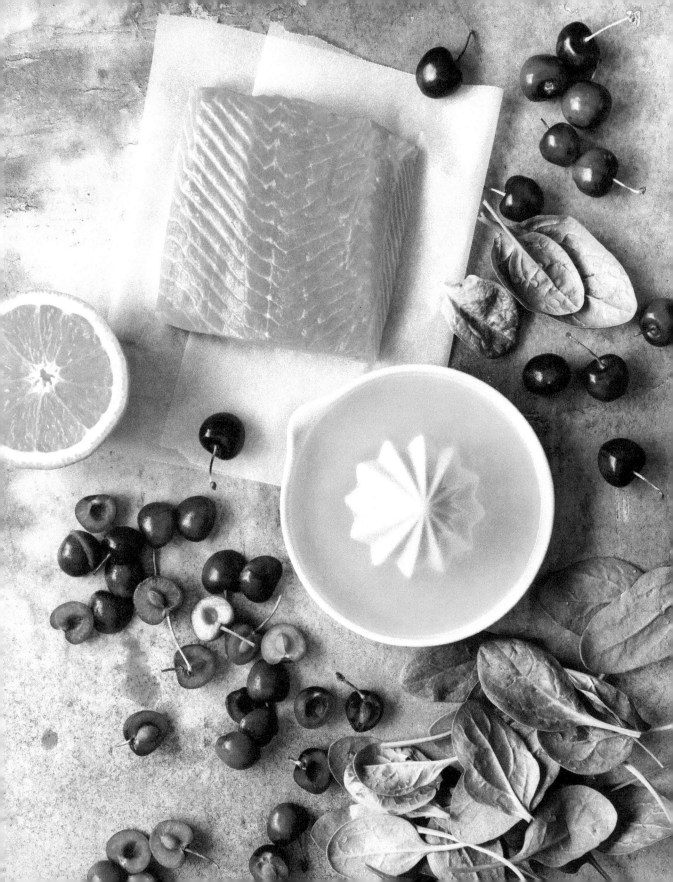

Gout is not a new disease. It is chronicled in medical periodicals as far back as 350 BC in the writings of Hippocrates. Credited as the "father of medicine," Hippocrates was one of the first to describe many diseases and medical conditions and focused on a natural approach to treating them. Historical accounts support that Hippocrates believed certain foods played a role in gout. Centuries later, gout continues to be simplified as a Victorian king's disease of affluence and overindulgence. Regrettably, conventional approaches to treating gout still persist. As medical practitioners, we need to remedy this outdated viewpoint and present gout as a common, contemporary condition that can be effectively treated with a combination of a healthy diet and lifestyle, as well as medication.

As a primary care physician and internist, I have not had a good book on gout to offer my patients—until now. One of the many things I enjoyed about *The 28-Day Gout Diet Plan* is that it has a modern, sophisticated approach to an ancient disease. Many patients are not well informed about diet except for the general advice to avoid alcohol and red meat. Sophia Kamveris offers current, concise, and evidence-based medical and nutritional information regarding gout. Rather than presenting the reader with what *not* to eat—which is often the case in trendy diet books—*The 28-Day Gout Diet Plan* presents a positive perspective of advising what the patient *can* eat. Her approach is not to deprive a person of enjoyable food because of a health condition, but to enrich them with recommendations to make favorable improvements in their diet and lifestyle. My gout patients struggle with trying to figure out how to structure meals and balance their diets. The strategic, gout-friendly menu plans and heart healthy recipes outlined in this book will ease and facilitate their efforts while promoting overall health and wellness.

This book also apprises readers of the medical implications and health outcomes of hyperuricemia. Managing uric acid levels is essential in helping to reduce the risk of a spectrum of metabolic conditions that can develop, which include hypertension, diabetes, and kidney disease. Implementing prudent, preventive dietary interventions can slow down the development of these comorbidities, especially diabetes.

Dr. William Osler—often regarded as the "father of modern medicine"—states, "Listen to your patient, he is telling you the diagnosis." Keeping an open line of communication with your physician is crucial. Education plays an integral role in a patient's treatment plan, and *The 28-Day Gout Diet Plan* reinforces the importance of building and fostering a relationship, and having an ongoing dialogue between patient and physician.

From a physician's perspective, I feel this book serves as a valuable and exceptional resource for gout sufferers. I will certainly recommend that my patients with high uric acid or gout heed Sophia's nutritional expertise and explore her joyful culinary creations presented in this well-designed, well-researched, and informative book. It's never too late to take charge of your health, and *The 28-Day Gout Diet Plan* is the definitive way to help you get started.

—**Arun Mukherjee, MD, MRCP, FACP**
Newton-Wellesley Physicians, Primary Care
An affiliate of Partners Healthcare

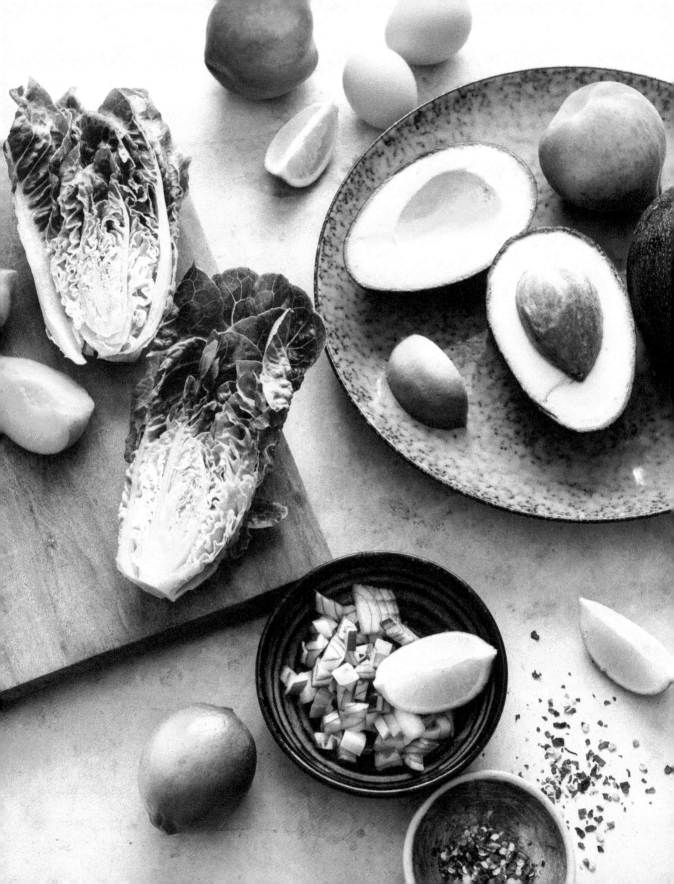

If you are reading this book, you or a loved one has gout. Purchasing this book means you have just made a significant investment in your healthy life. Not that I wish gout on anyone, but, if you're going to develop it, now is a good time. Thanks to decades-long research, we now have better insight into what gout is all about. You are not alone. Gout is on the rise globally, with a direct correlation to the prevailing increases in obesity, diabetes, and cardiovascular disease. Researchers report these conditions are a direct result of unhealthy lifestyle changes that include less exercise and 24/7 access to processed foods.

While there is no cure for gout, this book introduces you to the latest medical findings and gives you solid nutrition advice on what healthy foods to eat—both to avoid gout flares and decrease any long-term health risks associated with gout.

So, in addition to being a cookbook to help you (deliciously) manage gout, this is also a book with a bit of science tossed in to help you understand the condition better, leading to better self-care and disease management. Science helps us understand how our bodies work, and it's important to understand what makes gout tick.

I have been a registered dietitian for 35 years. I've seen a lot of diet trends, met with thousands of patients, and have counseled on countless diets in my career, but the one I was most apprehensive about was the low-purine diet. With trepidation I would enter a patient's hospital room to review the diet restrictions with them. As I read the list aloud, I would think to myself. "Who eats sweetbreads and meat

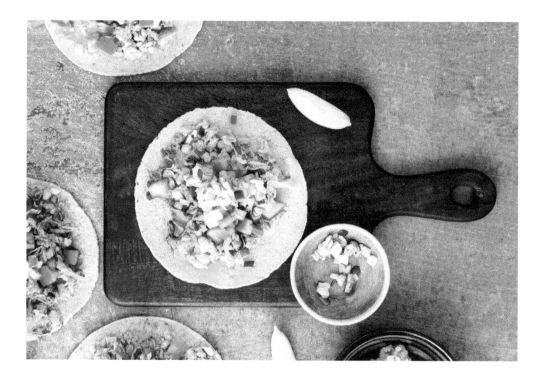

extracts?" I admit it now—I probably didn't do such a great job instructing them, mainly because I didn't really understand the disease or the diet very well myself.

Unlike some other medical conditions, gout really hurts. A patient shared that during a flare, the light wind from a fan blowing on his foot felt like an arrow piercing through it. Another was perplexed at how he went to bed feeling okay, and woke up wondering how he broke his ankle while sleeping.

As physically debilitating as gout is, it can also take an emotional toll and impact quality of life. People feel isolated at social gatherings because of their food restrictions, and many are reluctant to plan future activities, unsure how they will be feeling. The fear of the unknown adds anxiety to everyday living for some people. Sleep is disrupted, which leads to fatigue that affects work and home responsibilities. And many live in fear of an impending attack. Gout hurts physically and emotionally.

One of the more startling things I learned is that gout treatment plans have poor compliance rates as compared to other diseases. While it is the most medically well understood of all the diseases (we know its cause and how to treat it), it is the most misunderstood by patients. Education is a key component to gout management. It is a chronic disease but only seems to get everyone's attention when an acute attack occurs. Who wants to talk long-term treatment plans when your big toe won't stop throbbing?

The best time to talk with your health care provider is when you are not having an attack. They are your primary source of reliable, well-established medical information—not the internet. Schedule an appointment and talk long-term strategies. Education and implementing what you've learned take time, but it is vital to achieving success for long-term gout management.

This book is not intended to replace any advice given to you by your health care provider. Rather, it provides tools to help you comfortably communicate with them to ensure healthy outcomes now and in the future.

Everything you need to get started is at your fingertips. Meal planning, in general, can be a chore. Add to it the need to choose foods carefully and it can seem like a daunting task. So, I have designed a gout-friendly, 28-day meal plan with accompanying weekly shopping lists to relieve the burden and take the guesswork out of eating to manage your condition. I provide recipes that can be customized to fit different dietary needs. And in addition to day-to-day menu recommendations, you'll find simple and manageable strategies so you can enjoy dining out, vacation, and holiday experiences. You'll be covered from Week 1 through Week 4 with tips to help you through those challenging times we all encounter. On Week 5 and beyond, know that I am with you in spirit and you'll have all the tools you need for success.

Eating is one of life's greatest pleasures. It's time to take control and discover good food that has been scientifically proven to help manage gout, so you can get back to living your best life possible—pain free.

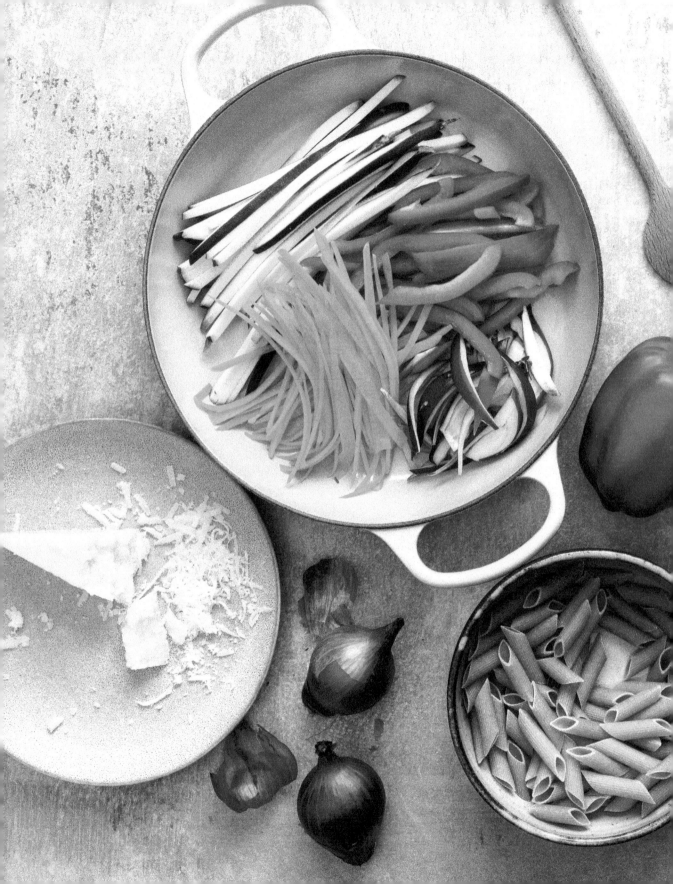

The Gout Diet and Meal Plan

Part One introduces you to the medical science of gout—how to treat it with medications and diet therapy, and the long-term medical risk factors. You'll also find a gout-friendly, 28-day meal plan designed to help lower uric acid levels, as well as helpful tips to manage day-to-day living, special occasions, vacations, and dining out.

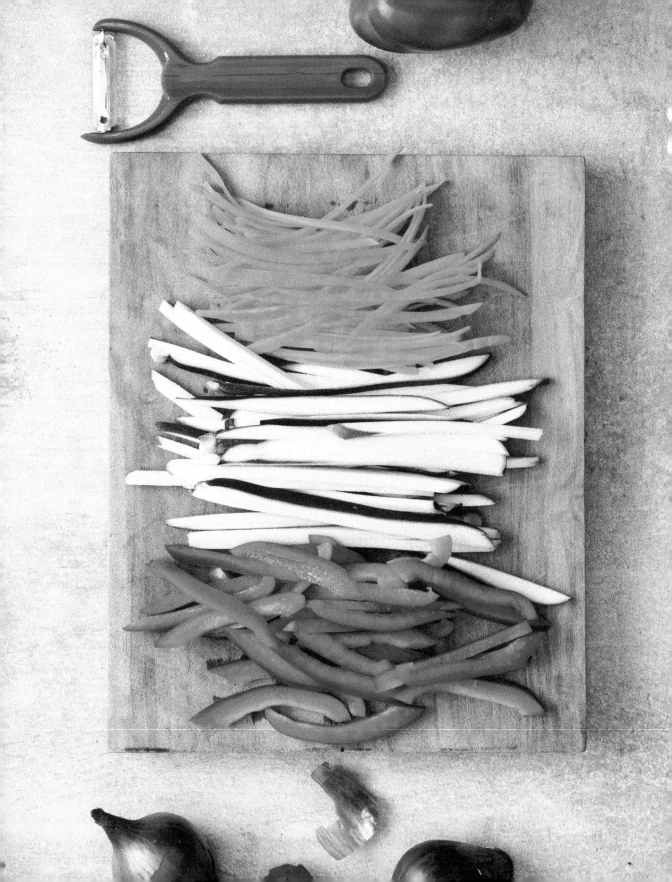

CHAPTER 1

Having a high uric acid level in your body is a predisposing factor for gout, and as far back as the mid-nineteenth century it had been determined that there is a direct relationship between elevated uric acid levels in the body, crystal formation in the joints, and developing gout. Chapter 1 introduces you to some scientific information; having solid knowledge about the medical component of this condition is critical for understanding how to manage gout effectively. No one with gout wants to experience the severe, disabling pain that a gout flare brings on, or live in fear of the next attack.

Long ago gout was touted as the disease of kings due to their overindulgence in rich food and wine. Today, it is the most common form of chronic inflammatory arthritis in men, ages 45 and older, and in postmenopausal women. Gout is characterized by a condition called hyperuricemia, which is an elevated level of uric acid in the blood. Left untreated, these high levels of serum uric acid deposit monosodium urate (MSU) crystals in the joints or around soft tissue. It's these needle-like crystals that cause pain and can debilitate people for weeks when they are having a gout attack. The disease presents itself as acute and episodic and results in severe pain, with a feeling of stiffness, heat, redness, and swelling in the afflicted joint. The most common site for a gout attack is the big toe, but it can also occur in an ankle, knee, heel, wrist, finger, or elbow. It can affect a single joint or multiple joints at one time.

Approximately one-third of the uric acid in the body comes from foods we eat; the remainder is inherently derived from our bodies. Uric acid is a compound produced in the liver from the breakdown of purines and is excreted primarily by the kidneys in our urine. Purine comes from the foods we eat and is also created by our bodies. Significant sources of dietary purine include animal organ meats such as sweetbreads, liver, and kidney; red meat; certain seafood; and beer and liquor. Purines are also natural and necessary substances found in our body that make up DNA and RNA—the basis of our body's genetic blueprint—and also play a significant role in how energy is produced in our bodies.

Uric acid crystals can also collect in the kidneys and form kidney stones. About 20 percent of gout patients will also develop kidney stones.

HYPERURICEMIA

You just learned that having abnormally high levels of uric acid in the blood is called *hyperuricemia*. These elevated levels occur either from the body producing too much uric acid, or the kidneys inadequately removing it from the body. Hyperuricemia itself is not a disease but it appears to be the main, if not the only, risk factor for gout. Years of epidemiological evidence supports a causal relationship between elevated uric acid levels in the blood and gout. These studies found that as serum uric acid rose, so did the relative risk for developing gout. That said, not all people with hyperuricemia will develop gout. In fact, up to two-thirds of people with hyperuricemia never develop symptoms.

Over the past few decades research studies have identified a rise in the prevalence of hyperuricemia and, by association, an increase in gout not only in the United States, but globally. According to the National Health and Nutrition Examination Survey (NHANES), 2007–2008, approximately 8.3 million people in the United States have gout. The evidence correlates a direct increase in uric acid levels to multiple factors that include changes in diet and lifestyle, a rise in medical conditions such as obesity, diabetes, hypertension, and kidney disease, as well as genetics, gender, and certain types of diuretic medications.

Hyperuricemia is commonly described as a "serum urate (another word for uric acid) concentration greater than 6.8 mg/dL." Above a certain uric acid threshold (greater than 6.8 mg/dL), monosodium urate crystals can begin to form and get deposited into joints. The goal is to maintain lower serum urate concentrations so fewer crystals are produced and deposited, which reduces gout flares.

Testing Uric Acid Levels

The blood test for uric acid is called serum uric acid (sUA) and is measured in milligrams per deciliter (mg/dL). Milligrams per deciliter is a measurement that indicates the amount of a particular substance in a specific amount of blood. In this case, it's the amount of uric acid in blood.

Issued by the American College of Rheumatology (ACR), the "2012 American College of Rheumatology Guidelines for Management of Gout" were developed using input from national and international medical experts. The guidelines recommend testing serum urate levels 2 weeks or more after a gout flare completely subsides. They also suggest regularly monitoring serum urate every 2 to 5 weeks during urate-lowering therapy, including continuing measurements every 6 months once the serum urate target is achieved. This gives practitioners a better perspective as to how compliant people are being with their medication, or if there is something else going on medically that needs to be addressed.

Keeping serum uric acid levels below 6 mg/dL helps reduce the likelihood of a gout attack. In people with greater disease severity, such as those with tophi (an accumulation of monosodium urate crystals), ACR recommends a serum urate level below 5 mg/dL to achieve better disease control.

THE STAGES OF GOUT

To gout sufferers, managing gout can seem like a full-time job. While some people might experience a sense of foreboding that a gout attack is imminent, others are hit out of the blue, most often at night.

The four stages of gout are classified according to the symptoms of the disease:

Stage 1: Asymptomatic hyperuricemia

Stage 2: Acute gouty arthritis

Stage 3: Intercritical gout

Stage 4: Chronic tophaceous gout

Each stage has its own protocol for managing, or at least minimizing, the physical pain and emotional stress while dealing with this chronic condition.

STAGE 1: ASYMPTOMATIC HYPERURICEMIA

Patients with asymptomatic hyperuricemia do not require treatment and may not even know they have it. *Asymptomatic*, by definition, means there are no symptoms of disease. Stage 1 is, essentially, a silent phase, as there are no obvious symptoms such as pain. But this is the time that MSU crystals begin to form and start to deposit in joints if serum urate concentrations exceed 6.8 mg/dL. These deposits can precede gout attacks, which can be triggered by the movement of crystals. Asymptomatic hyperuricemia can persist for many years without progression.

STAGE 2: ACUTE GOUTY ARTHRITIS

Symptoms of acute gouty arthritis, also known as acute gout, include excruciating pain, redness, warmth, and swelling in a joint. Gout flares or attacks most often begin at night while people are sleeping. The greatest severity of the flare occurs within 12 to 24 hours of onset. The attack can last from days to weeks and can resolve on its own. The goal of treatment in this stage is to provide prompt pain relief. Anti-inflammatory medications help control the pain and several studies have confirmed that an ice application to the joint helps as well.

Try to notice what may have set off an attack. Conditions such as a change in medication; diet or alcohol intake; trauma to a joint; surgery; dehydration; low body temperature; or low blood cortisol levels can all provoke a gout flare. Attacks can also occur with normal, or even low, serum urate concentrations at the time of the acute event. An interesting note is that serum uric acid levels tend to decrease during acute attacks. As the disease progresses, acute gout flares can become more frequent and may take longer to resolve.

STAGE 3: INTERCRITICAL GOUT

Once a gout attack resolves, one enters a symptom- and pain-free interval referred to as an intercritical ("between attack") period. There's no way to know how long this stage will last. It can be months or years before another gout attack occurs. It's important to understand that urate crystals may still be silently forming and depositing in your joints during this latent period.

This is an opportune time to talk with your health care provider to strategize and develop an individualized treatment plan that is manageable and that you can comply with long term. It's important to review your medication schedule and discuss ways to reduce uric acid levels to prevent future gout attacks.

Because diet is one way to keep uric acid levels under control, it's also the perfect time to meet with a registered dietitian to discuss lifestyle changes and focus on a healthy eating plan. The diet recommendations outlined in this book are designed to provide balance and variety and to encourage good eating patterns. The meal plans and recipes have been developed with the help of scientific studies that have proven which foods can help lower uric acid levels and keep gout flares at bay.

Dealing with Gout Flares

The sooner you treat the pain, the better. Getting treatment within the first 24 hours of the start of an attack can lessen its length and severity.

- Take over-the-counter anti-inflammatory medication immediately—but not aspirin, as it can worsen an attack.

- Call your health care provider to report the flare.

- Continue to take your gout medicine as prescribed.

- Apply ice to the affected joint for 20 to 30 minutes, several times a day, which can also help ease the pain.

- Elevate your joint for the next 24 hours and, if you must walk, use a cane to relieve additional pressure.

- Avoid tight clothing or socks.

- Drink a lot of fluids; aim for 8 to 16 cups of fluids a day, at least half being water (no alcohol or sweetened soda or juice).

- Relax, as stress can aggravate gout.

Know the flare will pass and that a combination of eating well, as prescribed in this book, and maintaining a healthy lifestyle can lessen the frequency of flare-ups.

STAGE 4: TOPHACEOUS GOUT

People who experience repeated gout flares or persistent hyperuricemia for many years can develop tophaceous gout. Chronic tophaceous gout is characterized by an accumulation of large numbers of densely packed urate crystals, or lumps, called tophi. They can take years to develop and may be calcified (hardened), but they are not painful. However, they can become inflamed and cause symptoms like those of a gout flare.

While tophi can be visible to the eye on a physical examination, pathology exams and imaging testing are more accurate methods to diagnose them. Tophi can be found in areas of the body with soft connective tissue, such as on ears, finger pads, tendons, bursae, joints, or ligaments. Tophi are distinctively characteristic of gout. The continued deposition of crystals can cause erosion of the bone and eventually progress to joint damage and a deformity called gouty arthropathy.

DIAGNOSIS

As gout is a form of arthritis, it shares some of the same symptoms as other arthritic conditions. What distinguishes it from the others, however, is that the joint pain and inflammation associated with gout can resolve on their own, and flare-ups are followed by a period with no symptoms. It's important to have an accurate diagnosis of gout before any medical treatment plan begins. A rapid and prompt diagnosis is also very important, as untreated gout can lead to other medical health risks (see page 12, Gout and Comorbid Diseases, for more information).

The gold standard for definitively diagnosing gout is a procedure called arthrocentesis, or joint aspiration. Fluid in the joint, known as synovial fluid, is removed from the affected joint capsule by a needle and syringe and examined under a microscope for the detection of monosodium urate (MSU) crystals. This is an invasive procedure and it doesn't give a thorough evaluation as to the extent of the crystal deposits that have occurred. It can also be painful. This test is usually recommended for new gout sufferers to get a baseline view to identify if crystals are present yet.

Alternatively, health care providers can diagnose gout using well-established diagnostic methods that include:

A physical examination: Your health care provider will ask how quickly the pain started, what medications you are taking, and what foods your diet includes.

Measuring uric acid levels in the blood: Remember, a high level of uric acid in your blood doesn't necessarily mean you have gout, just as a normal level doesn't mean you don't have it.

Prior medical history of gout, as well as any family member's personal medical history of gout. Recent advances in research have identified some genetic mutations that predispose a person to hyperuricemia, but have not conclusively determined the hereditary risk for gout.

Imaging studies, such as X-ray, ultrasonography, magnetic resonance imaging (MRI), and dual-energy computed tomography (DECT) scans, are especially useful to detect uric acid crystals in joints between flares.

YOUR MEDICAL TEAM

A multidisciplinary, integrated medical team approach offers the most effective treatment plan for managing gout. These health care professionals include your primary care physician, rheumatologist, and dietitian. Let's consider the role of each.

Primary Care Physician

A primary care physician is trained in internal medicine and has a continuing responsibility to oversee and provide a patient with a comprehensive medical treatment care plan. Your primary care physician is your first point of contact for the coordination of all your medical concerns. It's important to have a good level of communication with them, as research demonstrates an effective doctor-patient relationship plays an integral role in the quality of health care delivery.

Rheumatologist

A rheumatologist is a board-certified physician who specializes in the treatment of autoimmune and musculoskeletal (joint, muscle, bone) disorders commonly referred to as rheumatic diseases. In the case of gout, if uric acid levels are not improving and

Questions to Ask Your Doctor

Whether you are newly diagnosed or have chronic gout, your health care provider remains your principal source for reliable and accurate information regarding your medical condition. Here are some questions you can ask for optimizing communication.

What is gout?

What causes gout?

What are the symptoms of gout?

Can gout be cured?

Is gout genetic?

Is there a test for gout?

How is gout treated?

What is the long-term goal of gout therapy?

Is there a special diet to follow?

Are there any lifestyle changes to make?

Does losing weight help gout?

Do I have to stop drinking alcohol altogether?

Are there medications to prevent gout flares?

How do the medications work?

Do I have to take the medications for the rest of my life or just during an attack?

How often should I have blood work done?

What can I do to prevent another gout attack?

What do I do if I have a gout attack?

Can high uric acid levels have serious long-term consequences, and if so what can I do to prevent them?

What's the next step if I can't lower my uric acid levels?

Should I see a rheumatologist?

joint pain is not resolving, the primary care physician will refer you to a rheumatologist for their medical expertise and clinical evaluation. As experts in the treatment of arthritis, rheumatologists examine the patient to learn whether gout is the cause of their arthritis and will review medication treatment plans. The American College of Rheumatology guidelines denote criteria for when a referral to a rheumatologist is beneficial to act as a resource to primary care doctors.

As a member of the Academy of Nutrition and Dietetics, a Registered Dietitian (RD) or Registered Dietitian Nutritionist (RDN) has met the minimum academic and professional requirements to earn the RD or RDN credential and to distinctively qualify as a food and nutrition expert. A registered dietitian is highly trained and is the sole medically recognized expert in the field of nutrition to treat and prevent diseases.

Registered dietitians provide current, evidence-based nutrition practices to achieve healthy outcomes for specific medical conditions. They can prescribe a personalized menu plan to meet individual medical needs, and can teach you how to incorporate gout-, heart-, and kidney-friendly foods into your diet to maintain long-term health.

MEDICATION TO TREAT GOUT

The choice of medications used to treat gout relate directly to the stage of the disease (see page 5), as well as other medical conditions that include kidney disease, risk for bleeding, or history of a gastrointestinal ulcer. This section discusses the medication treatment plans for effective gout management. Many studies have reported very low rates of adherence to urate-lowering therapies (ULT) among gout sufferers. These therapies are an effective means of controlling hyperuricemia, and sticking with the medication treatment plan prescribed by your health care provider is proven to be the best way to prevent future gout attacks and minimize kidney damage. It's essential to understand that ULT treatment is lifelong.

First up are the best established medications prescribed for gout attacks with the primary goal of reducing pain. Anti-inflammatory medications are the best treatment for gout flares and should be started at the onset of a flare. This treatment is usually short term and limited to the duration of the flare. The most common anti-inflammatory agents for gout flares are:

- **Nonsteroidal anti-inflammatory drugs (NSAIDS),** such as naproxen and ibuprofen, which work to reduce swelling in a joint and quickly relieve the pain of an acute gout episode. They can shorten the length of an attack, especially if taken within the first 24 hours.

  Note: NSAIDS are contraindicated for patients with chronic kidney disease; you should not take NSAIDS if you suffer from chronic kidney disease. **Aspirin is not recommended to treat gout and can actually worsen symptoms.**

Glucocorticoids, also known as anti-inflammatory steroids, may be taken in pill form or by direct injection into an involved joint. These medications need to be tapered and should not be stopped abruptly without medical advisement. Prednisone is a common steroid given for gout.

Colchicine, a plant alkaloid, is derived from plants in the lily family, including meadow saffron and autumn crocus, and has been used to treat gout for more than 2,000 years. It has known gastrointestinal side effects.

Next are the first-line medications used for preventive long-term management of hyperuricemia. Their job is to maintain lower uric acid levels in the body. Reducing serum urate levels between flares is key to avoiding crystal formation and preventing gout attacks from occurring or reoccurring. They include the *uricostatic* agents that reduce the production of uric acid in your body, and are often referred to as XOIs (xanthine oxidase inhibitors). These include allopurinol, oxypurinol, and febuxostat.

Uricosuric agents, on the other hand, work by increasing the urinary excretion of uric acid by the kidneys. They include probenecid, benzbromarone, and the most recent—lesinurad.

It's important to note that some of these medications can temporarily trigger flares, but do not discontinue them without your physician's advice. New medications are in development as well, which have different target mechanisms.

GOUT AND COMORBID DISEASES

The definition of *comorbidity,* according to Merriam-Webster's dictionary, is a condition "existing simultaneously with and usually independently of another medical condition." This simply means that some medical conditions coexist with one another. The comorbidities of gout include hypertension and cardiovascular disease, chronic kidney disease, diabetes, obesity, and joint and bone disease. Many of these chronic diseases have a direct impact on uric acid levels in the body. As we already know, hyperuricemia is the number one risk factor for developing gout.

Effective treatment and better management of uric acid levels in gout is extremely important, not only to improve quality of life but also to ensure the reduction of these associated disease comorbidities.

Let's look at these medical conditions individually to further understand the reasons compliance with gout therapy is so crucial.

GOUT AND CHRONIC KIDNEY DISEASE

Almost 40 percent of patients with gout have chronic kidney disease. A symbiotic association exists between these two diseases. We know that gout results from the kidneys not excreting uric acid efficiently, allowing hyperuricemia to occur and uric acid crystals to form. Over time, these crystals can damage the kidneys, impairing kidney function. So, in this unique circumstance, kidney disease can lead to gout or gout can lead to kidney disease. According to the National Kidney Foundation, one in five people with gout will develop kidney stones—a product of uric acid. Left untreated, kidney stones can cause kidney infections and damage.

GOUT AND OBESITY

Excess weight can lead to diabetes and cardiovascular disease, putting people at a higher risk for gout. According to research studies, about 70 percent of people with gout are overweight and 14 percent are obese. Extra weight puts a strain on the kidneys, making it harder for them to remove uric acid. Studies have also shown that being obese increases your risk of developing gout sooner than someone of normal weight. Simply put, the more you weigh, the greater the risk of having recurrent gout attacks. Even a small amount of weight loss can lower uric acid levels.

GOUT AND CARDIOVASCULAR DISEASE

Research has indicated a causal relationship between hyperuricemia and cardio-vascular disease. Because of the potential effect high uric acid has on blood vessels, people with gout are twice as likely to suffer a heart attack or stroke as those without gout. Epidemiological data also show a connection between hyperuricemia and hypertension, demonstrating that a decrease in serum urate levels improves blood pressure control.

GOUT AND DIABETES

With diabetes, either your body doesn't produce enough insulin, the hormone that regulates the movement of sugar out of the blood and into the cells, or your body resists the effects of insulin, not letting it do its job to lower blood sugar. Elevated blood sugars (hyperglycemia) can damage blood vessels, which is a risk factor for developing cardiovascular and kidney disease. Uncontrolled diabetes can damage the eyes, kidneys, nerves, and blood vessels.

Insulin's primary role is to lower blood sugar. But when people are overweight or obese, cells become resistant to letting it in—a condition referred to as *insulin resistance.* Blood sugar levels remain elevated, tipping off the pancreas to produce more insulin. Now there's an elevated level of insulin circulating throughout the body, which can interfere with the kidneys' ability to excrete uric acid. The excess uric acid in the body can lead to gout and gout attacks.

GOUT AND JOINTS

We already know that hyperuricemia can lead to gout. Left untreated, progressive gout can be a long-term problem with permanent joint damage and constant pain. Gout symptoms can mimic the pain of another form of inflammatory arthritis called osteoarthritis (OA), which develops more slowly. A link has been established between gout and OA but further research is needed to understand the pathological relationship between the two. Being overweight is a common risk factor for gout and OA, so maintaining a healthy weight is important. Being overweight also adds more stress to the joints, causing more bone damage. A 2005 study of overweight and obese individuals with knee arthritis demonstrated that every one pound of excess weight exerts about four pounds of extra pressure on your knees. That means being 10 pounds overweight adds 40 pounds of extra pressure on the joint. Conversely, losing 10 pounds relieves 40 pounds of extra pressure on the joint—this relatively small amount of weight loss can greatly improve symptoms.

Tips for Successfully Managing Gout

While no cure exists for gout, making healthy lifestyle choices and maintaining medication compliance play key roles in how well it is controlled. With the right medicine, diet, and treatment plan, flares can be reduced and you can live pain free.

1. The first step to successfully managing gout is understanding fully what's at stake with this disease. One of the American College of Rheumatology's top recommendations is for more education on diet, lifestyle choices, treatment plans, and better medical management of comorbidities (see pages 12 to 14). This process begins with a conversation with your doctor and focuses on a comprehensive education plan that includes the importance of medication and diet compliance, and the long-term health risks associated with chronic uncontrolled hyperuricemia.

2. Diet is one critical component of managing gout, but taking your medication as prescribed by your health care provider is essential for keeping uric acid levels down. One research study reported that gout patients had the worst compliance rate for taking prescribed medications compared to other chronic conditions including hypertension, diabetes, thyroid disease, and high cholesterol. While you are the only one that can take your medications, studies show that social support from family, friends, or caregivers is important in helping people maintain good adherence practices to their prescribed medication and diet regimens.

3. Science tells us that comorbidities, like diabetes, cardiovascular disease, and chronic kidney disease, can develop over time from poorly managed gout. A 2015 European study of 3,079 gout patients found 68 percent had high blood pressure, 59 percent had high cholesterol, and 24 percent had type 2 diabetes. Unfortunately, some people view gout attacks as episodic—seeking treatment only for pain relief—and don't see the big picture when it comes to their overall health. This is most likely true of the asymptomatic hyperuricemia stage (see page 6) where there are no overt symptoms, but elevated uric acid levels can still exist, which increases the risk of developing health comorbidities.

4. The 28-day gout-friendly meal plan and recipes in this book are invaluable resources to help you start on the path to healthy living with gout. Eating a heart-healthy diet, exercising regularly, staying well hydrated, and watching your weight are important components of successful gout self-management.

5. After speaking with your health care provider, and with a more comprehensive understanding of gout, schedule an appointment with a registered dietitian. This nutrition expert will review your complete medical history, evaluate your food intake patterns, develop a personalized health plan, and offer lifestyle recommendations that are manageable and sustainable for long-term well-being.

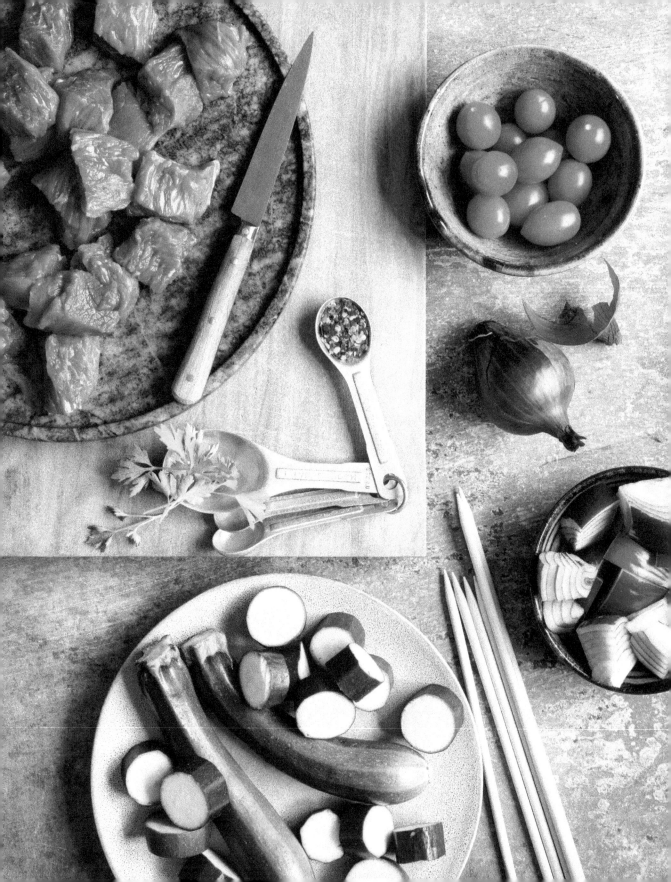

CHAPTER 2

The diet and lifestyle management tools for gout are not based on any popular diet trend. Instead, the dietary recommendations for gout are deeply rooted in decades of the best available research being conducted worldwide. This section addresses some of the latest epidemiological evidence that supports a whole food, nutrient-dense, heart-healthy approach to eating for managing gout. Remember, adopting healthy lifestyle habits sustainable for the long haul are the key components of an effective gout treatment plan.

NUTRITION AND TREATMENT OPTIONS

As we learned in chapter 1, the body breaks down purines into uric acid, and elevated uric acid levels can lead to gout. Rather than concentrate on purines solely as a causal factor for high uric acid levels, research has now identified which foods may actually help *lower* uric acid levels.

Fruits and vegetables are excellent sources of antioxidants, fiber, vitamins, and minerals that help our bodies stay in tiptop shape. Adding these nutrient-rich foods into your diet not only supports overall wellness, but recent evidence has shown that consuming a fruit and vegetable-based diet alkalinizes urine, increasing uric acid excretion, which naturally lowers uric acid levels and helps prevent gout attacks.

THE MOST RELIABLE NUTRITION RECOMMENDATIONS ARE BASED ON SCIENCE

The following diets have been proven to lower uric acid levels.

DASH Diet

Endorsed by the National Institutes of Health and American Heart Association, the Dietary Approaches to Stop Hypertension (DASH) diet has been proven to reduce blood pressure and prevent cardiovascular disease, which can accompany gout (see page 13). The good news for gout sufferers is the DASH diet may also help lower uric acid levels.

The DASH plan focuses on nutrient-dense whole foods that include low-fat dairy products, nuts and legumes, whole grains, heart-healthy fats, and fruits and vegetables. It also limits consumption of sodium, sweetened beverages, and red and/or processed meats. The dual role that DASH plays in gout—lowering blood pressure and uric acid levels—earns it an A+ rating. For this reason, 64 DASH-compliant recipes are included in this book.

Low-Purine Diet

Historically, conventional dietary recommendations for gout care have focused on restricting purine-rich foods. A decade-long study is shedding new light on this diet. Researchers now distinguish between animal and other protein sources of purine as it relates to hyperuricemia. The Health Professionals Follow-Up Study, which evaluated the influence of diet on illnesses, concluded that those participants with the highest meat and seafood intake—the top 20 percent—increased their risk of gout by almost 50 percent. The consumption of purine-containing vegetables, such as beans, lentils, mushrooms, and peas, did not affect uric acid levels.

As a result, the American College of Rheumatology (ACR) guidelines advise a limit on the serving sizes of red meat and seafood, while vegetables are unrestricted and encouraged as a part of a healthy menu plan. A recommended serving size of red meat and seafood is less than 6 ounces a day. All the recipes in this book are gout friendly, but some include moderate-purine foods like cod or haddock, clams, halibut, salmon, and shrimp as they provide great nutritional value in your diet.

Fructose, a naturally occurring sugar found in fruits, may also be linked to uric acid levels. As the body breaks down fructose, purines are released, leading to high serum uric acid levels. High-fructose corn syrup is a manmade sweetener produced from corn and composed of 55 percent fructose. For the past few decades, it has been found in abundance in commercially prepared baked goods, and especially in sweetened soft drinks. In one study, drinking sugar-sweetened soft drinks clearly increased the risk of gout in men, with a direct correlation to the volume consumed—the more they drank, the greater the risk for developing gout. Excess fructose also contributes to obesity, a known risk factor for gout. No recipes here use high-fructose corn syrup, but I have included fresh fruits, especially those that are significant sources of vitamin C and that have been proven to help lower uric acid levels naturally.

Why Is a Gout Diet So Hard to Manage?

Gout is a well understood disease but remains poorly managed for a variety of reasons. Misinformation gathered from the internet, from a person who knows someone with gout, from a waitress taking your order, or even from older physicians still treating gout with outdated medical modalities, all add to the complexities of managing gout. Many people also feel that diet alone can sufficiently manage their gout, but according to the American College of Rheumatology, diet changes may only yield a 10 to 18 percent drop in uric acid levels, which is not enough to dissolve crystals.

Obesity, hypertension, kidney disease, genetics, gender, not following doctor's orders, and side effects of some medications can also indirectly increase uric acid levels, making treating gout challenging for health care providers. Being properly educated on gout from a reliable medical source and having a very good working relationship with your health care provider are essential components of successful gout management.

FOOD: THE GOOD AND THE BAD

Popular, trendy diets often define themselves by the foods they omit, but a much healthier focus is incorporating a diversified, whole-foods approach to your eating. It's all about smart eating nowadays—just think of all the good foods you *can* eat instead of those you can't! The American College of Rheumatology recommendations have liberalized the diet. Making sensible food choices and applying moderation is key advice for maintaining a healthy, well-balanced diet.

HEALING FOODS

Including the following foods in your heart-healthy diet can help you manage your gout by lowering uric acid levels.

Cherries: Researchers in 1950 were the first to report on this fruit's positive impact on gout. Eating cherries restored serum uric acid levels to normal, and participants also reported less joint pain. Decades later, studies continue to support their health benefits. A recent study looked at the effects that eating fresh cherries or drinking cherry extract had over a two-day period; there was a 35 percent lower risk of gout attacks in the cherry group compared to the no-cherry group.

Researchers believe the antioxidant compound in cherries, anthocyanin, has anti-inflammatory properties and agree further studies are needed. For now, they are not discouraging the use of cherries in addition to physician-prescribed medications. I've included several recipes that incorporate the antioxidant power of cherries, but they can be added to any recipe or just eaten as a snack. So go ahead and start your day with a Juicy Cherry Smoothie (see page 52) or end it with Frozen Yogurt with Cherry Compote (see page 142) on top!

Vitamin C: This water-soluble vitamin helps build and repair cell tissues and has antioxidant properties that support a healthy immune system. Research now demonstrates it also has a protective effect against developing gout by increasing the renal excretion of uric acid by the kidneys. Some vitamin C–rich foods to add to your diet include dark green vegetables, tomatoes, potatoes, bell peppers, berries, guava, all citrus fruits, kiwi, papaya, and melon, which are used in abundance in the recipes in this book.

Water: Water is an essential nutrient that plays a vital role in our bodies—and especially in gout. The human body is largely made up of water and practically every cell in our body depends on it to function. As a main constituent of blood, water transports nutrients to cells all around the body, regulates body temperature (a flare trigger), and helps remove waste products that include uric acid (another flare trigger).

Lack of fluids plays a critical role in the development of uric acid crystals. Earlier we learned that dehydration can set off a gout flare; don't wait until you are thirsty to hydrate. To estimate how much water you should be drinking, divide your body weight (in pounds) by two, and aim to drink that many ounces of water every day.

Coffee and Low-Fat Dairy: Studies have also looked at the uric acid–lowering effect of coffee and low-fat dairy products. At this time, there are no formal recommendations other than they can be used as a part of a normal diet.

FOODS TO AVOID

The "2012 American College of Rheumatology Guidelines for Managing Gout" were developed over a two-year period by a special task force of national and internationally renowned experts. The guidelines are based on epidemiological evidence and outline specific recommendations that include medication, lifestyle, and dietary approaches to managing gout.

The guidelines' goals are to help manage the risk and frequency of acute gout attacks and address the best medical management practices to prevent gout-associated comorbidities, such as kidney disease and cardiovascular disease. They recommend weight loss, if obese; exercise; stopping smoking; and staying well hydrated, in addition to an overall heart-healthy diet for all individuals with gout.

The American College of Rheumatology dietary recommendations include:

AVOID	LIMIT	ENCOURAGE
Organ meats high in purine content (kidney, liver, sweetbreads)	Serving sizes of beef, lamb, pork	Low-fat or nonfat dairy products; vegetables
Any foods or beverages made with high-fructose corn syrup	Serving sizes of seafood with high purine content (sardines, shellfish)	
Any alcohol during a gout attack, or for anyone with poorly controlled, advanced gout	Serving sizes of naturally sweetened fruit juices	
	Table sugar and sweetened beverages and desserts	
	Table salt, including in sauces and gravies	
	Alcohol, particularly beer, but also wine and spirits; for men, limit to 2 servings per day; 1 serving per day for women	

THE TRIGGER-FREE KITCHEN

By now, you understand that the diet for gout management involves a whole-foods approach and includes more good-for-you foods. Having a well-stocked kitchen will ensure you eat smart and have the right foods available for creating delicious meals that are gout friendly and super healthy.

THE PANTRY

Some canned foods tend to be higher in sodium, especially soups, tomato products, and vegetables. Pay attention to the Nutrition Facts label and choose foods that have less than 10 percent of the Daily Value in sodium. Rinsing some foods can help remove some sodium, but purchase "no salt added" or low sodium if you can. Lowering sodium in your diet helps lower blood pressure and protect the kidneys, which work hard to eliminate uric acid.

Beverages

- Tart cherry juice
- Water: plain bottled; naturally flavored seltzer

Canned Goods

- Artichoke hearts packed in water
- Beans, low-sodium canned
- Broth, low-sodium chicken and vegetable (less than 140 mg of sodium per 8-ounce serving)
- Salmon, pouch, or low-sodium canned
- Tomato products, no-salt-added

Condiments, Oils, Vinegars

- Hot sauce: Louisiana-style, Frank's RedHot
- Mustard: Chinese hot, Dijon, or dried
- Oil: chili, extra-virgin olive, light olive, sesame
- Soy sauce, low-sodium
- Sriracha
- Vinegar: apple cider, balsamic, red wine, rice

Grains and Legumes

- Pearl barley
- Bread and hamburger rolls, whole-grain
- Bread crumbs, whole-wheat
- Flour, whole-wheat
- Lentils, dried
- Oats: old-fashioned rolled, steel-cut
- Pasta, whole-wheat
- Rice: brown, wild
- Tortillas: corn, whole-wheat

Nuts, Seeds, and Dried Fruit

- Dried fruit: apples, cherries, cranberries, raisins
- Nuts: unsalted; walnuts, pine nuts
- Nut butter: unsalted, all-natural
- Seeds: chia, flax, sesame

Spices and Sweeteners

- Black pepper
- Capers
- Cayenne pepper
- Chili powder
- Cilantro, fresh
- Cinnamon, ground
- Coriander, ground
- Cornstarch
- Cream of tartar
- Cumin, ground
- Curry powder
- Dill
- Extract: almond, vanilla
- Garlic powder
- Ginger, fresh
- Honey
- Italian seasoning
- Maple syrup, pure
- Mrs. Dash, any blend you prefer, or other salt-free seasonings
- Oregano
- Red pepper flakes
- Rosemary
- Sage
- Salt: kosher and sea
- Sugar, brown, granulated
- Tarragon
- Thyme
- Turmeric, fresh root and ground
- Unsweetened cocoa powder

THE REFRIGERATOR

Studies have found that the use of low-fat dairy helps reduce uric acid levels, so keep your refrigerator well stocked with these items. If you have dairy allergies, there are a variety of milk substitutes commercially available, but these have not been proven to have an effect on uric acid levels.

The Gout-Free Food Recommendations

So far, we have learned that gout is caused by a mix of genetics, lifestyle, and environmental factors, and that having gout puts you at risk for developing other medical conditions, or comorbidities. Obviously, two risk factors—gender and genetics—are out of your control. Otherwise, you are pretty much in the driver's seat regarding setting the course of this disease. By implementing the tools provided in this book—well-established medical information, a 28-day meal plan, and easy-to-use recipes—you will be cruising down the road in no time, enjoying a healthy eating plan you can comfortably manage.

There are fundamental strategies that promote healthy eating patterns for everyone. They aim for balance and variety, and emphasize heart-healthy recommendations—we all want a strong ticker! Healthy fats; whole fruits and vegetables; leaner cuts of meats, poultry, and fish; nuts; and complex carbohydrates that include whole grains and legumes should all be staples in your diet. The meal plan and recipes included in this book are designed with these key nutrients in mind. Let's see how easily they fit into a gout-friendly diet plan.

Sodium for Heart and Kidney Health

Both the American Heart Association and the DASH diet recommend limiting sodium to approximately 2,300 milligrams per day. That's the amount of sodium in 1 teaspoon of salt. Controlling blood pressure helps the kidneys work more efficiently. Use more spices and herbs to season foods and cook with less salt. The recipes here burst with flavors from lemons and limes, which are packed with vitamin C. Processed foods, such as canned soups, deli meats, and frozen prepared meals, tend to be quite high in sodium, so pay attention to food labels. Always choose the lower-sodium option.

Fat for Heart Health and Anti-inflammatory Benefits

The American Heart Association (AHA) and the DASH diet also recommend limiting saturated fats, such as palm oil, palm kernel oil, and coconut oil, as they raise LDL (bad) cholesterol. Avoid trans fats and partially hydrogenated oils altogether. Choose heart-healthy polyunsaturated fats such as sunflower, sesame, or safflower oils and monounsaturated fats such as olive oil, nuts, and avocados. These types of fats help improve your cholesterol levels. Omega-3 fatty acids, found in cold-water fish, seeds, and nuts also help lower the risk of heart disease and reduce inflammation through-out the body. The AHA recommends eating fish at least twice a week to reduce cardiovascular risk. Whitefish has a lower purine content and is a good choice to include in your diet, for both gout and heart disease.

Sugar for Weight, Blood Sugar, and Uric Acid Control

Consumption of excess sugar has been linked to poor health conditions that include obesity, diabetes, and metabolic syndrome—all comorbidities for gout. Concentrated sources of sugar, such as candy, soft drinks, and baked goods, raise blood sugars quickly, triggering an insulin response that can elevate uric acid levels.

Choosing complex carbohydrates that are digested more slowly will keep blood sugars in check. These include whole grains, legumes, fresh fruits, and vegetables.

Limit your intake of added sugars from sweets and sugary beverages.

Balance for Weight Management

Excess weight negatively affects the body's ability to function efficiently. Losing weight helps keep blood sugars down and improves insulin sensitivity. It controls blood pressure, and that means less strain on the kidneys. Obesity promotes hyper-uricemia, while weight loss leads to a reduction in uric acid levels. Keeping your weight within a normal BMI level (less than 25) is a healthy goal.

Dairy, Eggs, Dairy Substitutes	Fruits and Vegetables	Beef, Pork, Fish, Poultry
Cheese: blue, feta, Monterey Jack, mozzarella, Parmesan, pepper Jack	Avocado	Canadian bacon
	Bell peppers	Fish: cod, flounder, haddock, halibut, salmon (wild or farmed)
Eggs	Cherries, in season	Pork tenderloin
Greek yogurt, plain low-fat	Citrus: lemons, limes, oranges	Poultry: low-fat cuts such as skinless chicken or turkey breast, or ground turkey or chicken breast; turkey sausage
Milk, low-fat	Garlic	
Orange juice	Green vegetables: bok choy, broccoli, kale, spinach, Swiss chard	
Tofu, extra firm	Onions: shallots, scallions	Red meat, lean cuts such as flank, tenderloin, sirloin
	Pomegranate	
	Sweet potatoes	

THE FREEZER

Having a well-stocked freezer as a backup to those hectic days when you aren't able to stop at the grocery store is a lifesaver! I'm always asked whether frozen fruits and vegetables are as healthy as fresh. The answer is yes, and frozen may even surpass the nutritional quality of fresh. Just-picked, farm-fresh produce is loaded with nutrition and should be your first choice. But the longer produce is in transit or stays on the supermarket shelf, the more nutrients are lost. Once fruits and vegetables are picked, they sit in a warehouse before they are hauled into a truck to be delivered to a grocery store and then finally make it into your refrigerator. Conversely, when fruits and veggies are harvested for commercial freezing, they are picked when fully ripe—at their nutritional peak. So, if you can't eat just-picked produce, frozen is the next best thing.

Berries: blackberries, blueberries, cherries, strawberries	Frozen yogurt, low-fat	Pancakes or waffles, whole-grain
	Lean red meats: see "Beef, Pork, Fish, Poultry" (page 26)	
Fish: see "The Refrigerator" (page 23)		

COOKING EQUIPMENT

It would be nice to have all the fancy kitchen gadgets a professional chef has to whip up a meal, but having the fundamentals on hand works just fine. Some tools do speed up the preparation process, and the quicker the better is an added benefit for our hectic lives. Lack of counter or storage space and cost are certainly considerations. And there's nothing wrong with cooking the old-fashioned way. Our grandparents managed just fine!

Essentials

- 9-inch square baking pan
- 10- or 12-inch nonstick skillet
- 12-cup muffin tin
- Baking sheet
- Blender
- Grater
- Pots, assorted sizes
- Saucepan
- Slow cooker

Measuring

- Liquid measuring cup
- Set of dry measuring cups
- Set of measuring spoons

Mixing and Cutting

- Knives: chef's, paring
- Mixing bowls: small, medium, and large
- Silicone scraper
- Spatula
- Whisk
- Wooden spoon

Miscellaneous

- Mason jars, small
- Parchment paper
- Ramekins
- Vegetable peeler
- Wooden skewers
- Zester

Nice to Have

- Apple peeler and corer
- Citrus juicer
- Food processor
- Indoor or outdoor grill
- Stove-top grill pan

When You Have Gout but the Rest of the Family Doesn't

Today, no one with gout should feel like a castaway stranded on an island with limited access to food options. As gloomy as the purine-restricted diet may seem, studies have demonstrated that family members feel guilty about eating different foods than their loved ones with gout. What should be enjoyable family time can potentially turn into an unpleasant dining experience.

The good news is the most up-to-date science has loosened the parameters of the traditional purine diet. Now, there's more flexibility with food choices and you are welcomed (and encouraged!) to eat like the rest of the family . . . but, this isn't a free pass to overindulge. You need to make sound and sensible decisions when it comes to eating. Eat fewer processed convenience and fast foods, pay attention to portion sizes, and choose the healthy foods as laid out for you in this book.

THE RECIPES

I have taken the latest medical science and combined it with some of Mother Nature's best offerings to develop a bountiful variety of gout-friendly, cook-friendly, and heart-healthy recipes designed to help lower uric acid levels and manage your weight. What's better than good recipes? Recipes that are good for you!

TYPES OF DISHES

People live busy lives these days so these recipes are designed to not only be gout-friendly and nutritious, but also easy to prepare. And because a good meal doesn't have to break the bank, these recipes call for simple, affordable ingredients. Most of these delicious meals are ready in 30 minutes—start to finish. I also include some new flavors. Treat yourself to some scrumptious dishes that are easy to make and yummy to eat. You deserve it!

HELPFUL LABELS

Throughout the book, I stress the importance of healthy eating because of the impact gout has on your kidneys, heart, and weight over the long haul. I kept all these precious body parts in mind while developing the recipes, incorporating the foods that help lower uric acid levels naturally. At the top of each recipe, you'll find labels that identify the diets the recipe complies with, making it easier to select the ones for your specific medical needs. **All recipes in this book are DASH Diet friendly.** This lifelong approach to healthy eating, including whole grains, fruits, vegetables, legumes, and low-fat dairy and limiting sodium to 2,300 mg per day, offers variety and flexibility to everyday menu planning and helps control blood pressure and weight. **All recipes in this book are also Heart Healthy.** Eating well for heart health is important to everyone who wants a strong ticker! The American Heart Association recommends no more than 5 to 6 percent of total calories come from saturated fat. Based on 2,000 calories a day, that's 13 grams per day.

- **Diabetes Friendly:** The DASH eating pattern can be helpful in managing diabetes. The plan focuses on using more plant-based foods like fresh fruits and vegetables, whole grains, nuts, seeds, and legumes, as well as lean protein, fish, and low-fat dairy products. Highly processed, refined grains and sugar-sweetened beverages are not recommended.

- **Gluten Free:** You'll be covered if you have celiac disease or are gluten sensitive.

- **Kidney Friendly:** It's important to take stress off those workhorse organs by watching out for excess sodium and potassium (the American Kidney Foundation recommends limiting both to 2,000 mg per day), and moderating protein in your diet.

- **Vegan/Vegetarian:** Following vegetarian (including eggs, dairy, and honey) and vegan (no animal by-products or honey included) diets helps lower blood pressure and reduces the risk of developing heart disease and type 2 diabetes.

TIPS

Whether you are a pro in the kitchen or are just learning your way around, you can make these recipes. Expert culinary tips are included with each recipe to offer recommendations to simplify, modify, or diversify a recipe. I have also included some nutrition education regarding the key nutrients that not only make these recipes healthy for you, but also are major players in helping lower your risk of a gout attack and in lessening the inflammation that accompanies such an attack.

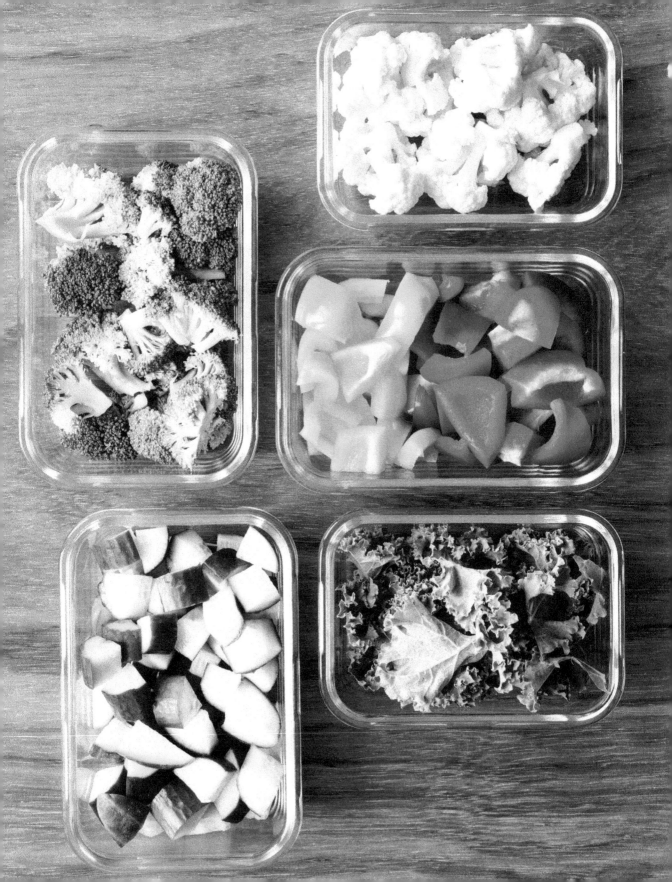

CHAPTER 3

T he fun is about to begin! It's all about the good foods you eat from now on. This chapter puts everything together for you—shopping lists, meal plans, recipes, cooking and preparation pointers, snacking suggestions, and dining-out, vacation, and holiday tips. Toss the takeout menus! Your kitchen will be sizzling with healthy meals you prepare and personally deliver to your dining room table every day. Unfurl the tablecloth because you'll be serving up some fun and flavorful foods this month!

WEEK 1

Starting anything new can be overwhelming but if you've got your eye on the prize, it's all worth it in the end. I know that trying new foods can be intimidating, but once you see how good healthy food can taste and how easy it is to prepare, you will be on your way to feeling great. This 28-day plan will take the guesswork out of meal planning and is designed so there's no cooking at breakfast or lunch Monday through Friday— but be ready for some extra preparation on the weekends. This book will provide all the fundamental tools you need to make this a healthful and successful venture. So, enjoy the ride. We are on this journey together!

WEEK 1 MEAL PLAN

	BREAKFAST	LUNCH	DINNER	SNACKS AND DESSERT
Sunday	Salmon and Kale Scramble (page 61)	Chicken Zoodle Soup with White Beans (page 66)	Spaghetti with Chicken Meatballs and Marinara (page 94)	Choose one or two snacks each day from the snack list provided below, and treat yourself to some homemade, yummy desserts this week!
Monday	Juicy Cherry Smoothie (page 52)	Spaghetti with Chicken Meatballs and Marinara (leftovers)	Sirloin Tips with Mushrooms and Brown Rice (page 114)	Veggie sticks with 2 tablespoons hummus or ¼ cup low-fat yogurt dip
Tuesday	Slow-Cooker Fruit 'n' Oats (page 54)	Salmon and Arugula Salad with Blackberry Vinaigrette (page 70)	Lemon Pepper Cod with Lemony Sautéed Greens (page 128)	3 cups unsalted popcorn 1 cup melon chunks, grapes, berries, or cherries 1 small piece of fruit
Wednesday	Honeyed Orange Pomegranate Yogurt (page 53)	Chicken Zoodle Soup with White Beans (leftovers)	Black Bean and Veggie Burritos (page 79)	3 pieces of dried fruit (especially cherries; apricots, prunes, dates)
Thursday	Slow-Cooker Fruit 'n' Oats (leftovers)	Chopped Italian Salad (page 71)	Asian Ground Turkey and Bok Choy Stir-Fry (page 93)	¾ cup low-fat milk with 2 graham cracker squares 10 unsalted almonds or 2 whole walnuts
Friday	Juicy Cherry Smoothie (page 52)	Asian Apple and Cabbage Slaw with Roasted Chicken (page 69)	Thin-Cut Pork Chops with Gingered Applesauce (page 112)	5 ounces low-fat vanilla Greek or Icelandic-style yogurt 4 whole-grain crackers and 1 ounce low-fat Cheddar or string cheese
Saturday	Red Bell Pepper Omelet (page 60)	Tuscan Bean, Kale, and Turkey Sausage Soup (page 64)	Salmon with Ginger-Cherry Sauce and Spinach (page 132)	4 whole-grain crackers with 2 tablespoons hummus or 1 tablespoon all-natural peanut butter

WEEK 1 SHOPPING LIST

Eggs and Dairy

Eggs, large, 1½ dozen

Cheese, shredded Monterey Jack, ¼ cup

Cheese, shredded mozzarella, 2 ounces (½ cup)

Cheese, shredded pepper Jack, ½ cup

Milk, low-fat, ½ gallon

Yogurt, plain low-fat Greek, 1 quart

Produce

Apples, sweet-tart, 5

Baby arugula, 4 cups

Basil, fresh, 1 bunch

Bell peppers, red, 3

Bing cherries, fresh, 2 cups; and frozen, 1½ cups

Blackberries, fresh, ¼ cup

Bok choy, 1 head

Cabbage, 1 large head, or 1 (14-ounce) bag coleslaw mix

Carrot, 1

Celery, 1 bunch

Cilantro, 1 bunch

Cremini mushrooms, 8 ounces

Cucumber, 1

Dried fruit of choice,1 cup

Garlic, 3 large heads

Ginger, fresh, 2 (5- to 6-inch) pieces

Jalapeño pepper, 1

Kale, 2 bunches

Lemons, 3

Limes, 3

Onions, 4

Oranges, 6

Parsley, 1 bunch

Pomegranate, 1 or pomegranate arils (seeds), ½ cup

Red onion, 1

Scallions, 1 bunch

Shallots, 4

Spinach, 4 cups

Tomatoes, cherry, 2 cups

Tomato, small, 1

Zucchini, large, 2

Canned Goods and Pantry Items

Artichoke bottoms (packed in water), no-salt-added, 1 (14-ounce) can

Black beans, low-sodium, 1 (15.5-ounce) can

Bread crumbs, whole-grain, 1 container

Chicken broth*, low-sodium, 3 quarts

Oats, steel-cut, 1 container

Rice, brown, 1 box

Spaghetti, whole-wheat, 1 box

Tomatoes, no-salt-added, diced, 1 (15.5-ounce) can

White beans, low-sodium, 2 (15.5-ounce) cans

*Note: If you plan to make homemade Poultry Broth (page 148), refer to the recipe and adjust this shopping list accordingly.

Packaged Goods

Pecans, chopped, ¼ cup

Pine nuts, ¼ cup

Salmon, wild-caught, 2 (5-ounce) pouches

Bread and Bread-Like Products

Tortillas, whole-wheat, 4

Beef, Pork, Fish, Poultry

Beef sirloin tips, 12 ounces

Canadian bacon, 3 ounces

Chicken breast, boneless, skinless, 8 ounces

Chicken breast, cooked, chopped, 2 cups

Chicken breast, ground, 12 ounces

Cod fillets, 4 (3-ounce)

Sausage, Italian turkey, 8 ounces

Pork chops, thin-cut, 4

Salmon fillets, 4 (3-ounce)

Turkey breast, 93% lean ground, 12 ounces

WEEK 1 TIPS

Even though I provide weekly grocery lists, it's a good idea to scan the recipes before you shop each week. Make sure to check the dates on perishable items you purchase, especially meat and seafood.

Your kitchen should be stocked with the nonperishable ingredients listed in the pantry list (see page 22); these items will be used over the course of the month. Some spices may be new to you, but I promise they offer a blend of delicious flavors at each meal!

Dinners are prepared nightly, while breakfast and lunch are prepped on the weekend. A slow cooker is used for some recipes (this week it's steel-cut oats) to help you out. I have designed the menu to start on Sunday, so you can prep for the week ahead. Plan to shop on Saturday and cook on Sunday.

Since this is your first week, it's okay to take some shortcuts and purchase a cooked rotisserie chicken for the luncheon salads. Low-sodium chicken broth is readily available on store shelves, and shredded cabbage (coleslaw mix) is in the produce section of the grocery store.

Looking ahead to this week:

On Sunday:

- Cook the steel-cut oats. The oatmeal can be refrigerated for up to 1 week, or it can be frozen.

- Prepare the blackberry and Asian vinaigrettes, which can be refrigerated for up to 3 days and 1 week, respectively. There is no substitution for taste when it comes to fresh ingredients and bottled dressings are loaded with salt and sugar.

- You can use packaged wild-caught salmon for the arugula salad.

- Remember to limit servings of meat and seafood to less than 6 ounces per day.

WEEK 2

With Week 1 behind you—congratulations!—you are likely getting into the swing of things. Organizing your lunch might be a new habit you're developing, but planning ahead means the difference between a healthy meal (and your health!) and that not-so-healthy fast-food drive-through. Invest in storage containers that can accommodate leftovers and pack your lunch after dinner to save time in the morning. Also, eat at the table, without any distractions (that means putting away the electronics!) so you can enjoy your meal. Slow down and give yourself plenty of time to eat. Remember, it takes 15 minutes for your brain and stomach to communicate with one another.

WEEK 2 MEAL PLAN

	BREAKFAST	LUNCH	DINNER	SNACKS AND DESSERT
Sunday	Tomato and Spinach Frittata (page 56)	Open-Faced Turkey Burger Caprese (page 73)	Flank Steak Chimichurri with Grilled Vegetables (page 118)	Choose one or two snacks each day from the snack list provided below, and treat yourself to some homemade, yummy desserts this week!
Monday	Spiced Apple Walnut Overnight Oats (page 55)	Salmon and Arugula Salad with Blackberry Vinaigrette (page 70)	Turkey with Wild Rice and Kale (page 92)	Veggie sticks with 2 tablespoons hummus or ¼ cup low-fat yogurt dip
Tuesday	Juicy Cherry Smoothie (page 52)	Tuscan Bean, Kale, and Turkey Sausage Soup (page 64)	Bell Pepper and Tofu Stir-Fry (page 80)	3 cups unsalted popcorn
				1 cup melon chunks, grapes, berries, or cherries
Wednesday	Tomato and Spinach Frittata (leftovers)	Spinach, Walnut, and Strawberry Salad with Citrus Vinaigrette (page 68)	Almond-Crusted Salmon with Green Beans (page 131)	1 small piece of fruit
				3 pieces of dried fruit (especially cherries; apricots, prunes, dates)
				¾ cup low-fat milk with 2 graham cracker squares
Thursday	Spiced Apple Walnut Overnight Oats (leftovers)	Bell Pepper and Tofu Stir-Fry (leftovers)	Chicken Satay with Peanut Sauce (page 102)	10 unsalted almonds or 2 whole walnuts
Friday	Honeyed Orange Pomegranate Yogurt (page 53)	Chopped Italian Salad (page 71)	Steamer Clams with Lemon Fennel Broth (page 125)	5 ounces low-fat vanilla Greek or Icelandic-style yogurt
				4 whole-grain crackers and 1 ounce low-fat Cheddar or string cheese
Saturday	Black Bean Breakfast Burrito (page 58)	Buffalo Chicken Wrap (page 72)	Pork Tenderloin Fajitas with Guacamole (page 110)	4 whole-grain crackers with 2 tablespoons hummus or 1 tablespoon all-natural peanut butter

WEEK 2 SHOPPING LIST

Eggs and Dairy

Cheese, crumbled blue,
2 tablespoons

Cheese, grated
Parmesan, ¼ cup

Cheese, shredded low-fat
Cheddar, ½ cup

Cheese, shredded
mozzarella, 1 cup

Eggs, large, 1 dozen

Milk, low-fat, 1 quart

Yogurt, low-fat plain
Greek, 1 quart

Produce

Avocados, 2

Baby arugula, 4 cups

Baby spinach, 6 cups

Basil, 1 bunch

Bell peppers, green, 2

Bell peppers, orange, 1

Bell peppers, red, 3

Bing cherries, fresh or
frozen, 1½ cups

Blackberries, fresh, ¼ cup

Carrots, 3

Cilantro, 1 bunch

Cucumber, 1

Fennel, 1 bulb

Garlic, 3 large heads

Ginger, fresh, 1 (6-inch) piece

Green beans, 2 cups

Jalapeño peppers, 2

Kale, 1 bunch

Lemons, 3

Limes, 8

Oranges, 3

Onions, 3

Parsley, Italian, 1 bunch

Pomegranate, 1, or
pomegranate arils
(seeds), ½ cup

Red onion, 2

Scallions, 1 bunch

Shallots, 4

Strawberries,
1 (1-pound) package

Tomatoes, cherry, 3 cups

Tomato, large, 1

Zucchini, 1

**Canned Goods and
Pantry Items**

Almond meal, 1 bag

Artichoke bottoms (packed
in water), no-salt-added,
1 (14-ounce) can

Black beans, low-sodium,
1 (15.5-ounce) can

Chicken broth*, low-sodium,
2 quarts

Coconut milk, lite, 1
(14-ounce) can

Oats, old-fashioned, rolled,
1 container

Peanut butter, all-natural,
no-salt-added, ½ cup

Tomatoes, no-salt-added,
diced, 1 (14-ounce) can

White beans, low-sodium,
1 (15.5-ounce) can

Wild rice, ¾ cup uncooked

*Note: If you plan to make
homemade Poultry Broth
(page 148), refer to the recipe
and adjust this shopping list
accordingly.

Packaged Goods

Dried apples, ½ cup

Pine nuts, ¼ cup

Salmon, wild-caught,
1 (5-ounce) pouch

Walnuts, chopped ½ cup
plus 2 tablespoons

**Bread and Bread-Like
Products**

Bread, whole-wheat, 1 loaf

Tortillas, whole-wheat, 10

Beef, Pork, Fish, Poultry

Beef flank steak, 12 ounces

Canadian bacon, 3 ounces

Chicken breast, boneless,
skinless, 18 ounces

Chicken breast, cooked,
chopped, 1 cup

Clams, steamer or Manila,
3 pounds

Pork tenderloin, 12 ounces

Salmon fillets, 4 (3-ounce)

Sausage, Italian turkey,
8 ounces

Turkey breast, 93% lean
ground, 24 ounces

Miscellaneous

Tofu, extra firm, 12 ounces

WEEK 2 TIPS

Before you head out shopping for this week's groceries, review the meal plan and recipes for Week 2. Check your refrigerator for any foods you can use this week—milk, yogurt, parsley, fresh ginger, garlic, onions, etc. Leftover vegetables can also be used in soups and stir-fries—I don't want you to waste any food! Refer to the recipes for which meals can be frozen, as well.

All recipes indicate serving sizes, so adjust accordingly based on your family size, or if you want to make extra to freeze for leftovers.

Remember to keep red meat and seafood portions to less than 6 ounces (cooked) per serving and include water at every meal and in between. No sugar-sweetened soft drinks! Staying hydrated helps keep the uric acid from crystalizing and staves off a gout attack.

Looking ahead to Week 2's meal preparation:

On Sunday:

Prepare the blackberry and citrus vinaigrettes, which can be refrigerated for up to 3 days and 5 days respectively.

On Thursday:

Save 1 cup of cooked chicken from Thursday night's dinner (before it is mixed with the peanut sauce) for Friday's lunch.

Purchase the clams for Friday's dinner.

WEEK 3

You're over the hump and by now may be noticing an extra pep in your step from all the good food you are feeding your body! Are you still on course? I know slipups happen; when they do, brush them off and get back on track. Make sure you get enough sleep. Fatigue can lead to overeating. And, sometimes when you think you are hungry, you are actually dehydrated! So, the next time you feel hungry drink a glass of water first.

WEEK 3 MEAL PLAN

	BREAKFAST	LUNCH	DINNER	SNACKS AND DESSERT
Sunday	Red Bell Pepper Omelet (page 60)	White Bean Chili (page 81)	Hearty Meat Loaf Muffins (page 113)	Choose one or two snacks each day from the snack list provided below, and treat yourself to some homemade, yummy desserts this week!
Monday	Slow-Cooker Fruit 'n' Oats (page 54)	Asian Apple and Cabbage Slaw with Roasted Chicken (page 69)	Sweet-and-Sour Tofu and Veggie Stir-Fry (page 84)	· Veggie sticks with 2 tablespoons hummus or ¼ cup low-fat yogurt dip
Tuesday	Black Bean Breakfast Burrito (leftovers from previous week)	Hearty Meat Loaf Muffins (leftovers)	Roasted Halibut with Tropical Black Bean Salsa (page 130)	· 3 cups unsalted popcorn · 1 cup melon chunks, grapes, berries, or cherries
Wednesday	Juicy Cherry Smoothie (page 52)	Sweet-and-Sour Tofu and Veggie Stir-Fry (leftovers)	Thin-Cut Pork Chop with Gingered Applesauce (page 112)	· 1 small piece of fruit · 3 pieces of dried fruit (especially cherries; apricots, prunes, dates)
Thursday	Honeyed Orange Pomegranate Yogurt (page 53)	White Bean Chili (leftovers)	Balsamic Chicken Breast with Brussels Sprouts (page 90)	· ¾ cup low-fat milk with 2 graham cracker squares
Friday	Slow-Cooker Fruit 'n' Oats (leftovers)	Buffalo Chicken Wrap (page 72)	Baked Fish and Chips with Tartar Sauce (page 126)	· 10 unsalted almonds or 2 whole walnuts · 5 ounces low-fat vanilla Greek or Icelandic-style yogurt
Saturday	Salmon and Kale Scramble (page 61)	Minestrone Soup (page 65)	Slow-Cooker Turkey Breast with Root Vegetables (page 98)	· 4 whole-grain crackers and 1 ounce low-fat Cheddar or string cheese · 4 whole-grain crackers with 2 tablespoons hummus or 1 tablespoon all-natural peanut butter

WEEK 3 SHOPPING LIST

Eggs and Dairy

Buttermilk, low-fat, 1 cup

Cheese, crumbled blue,
2 tablespoons

Cheese, shredded low-fat
Cheddar, ½ cup

Cheese, shredded Monterey
Jack, ½ cup

Eggs, large, 2 dozen

Milk, low-fat, 1 quart

Yogurt, plain low-fat
Greek, 2 cups

Produce

Apples, sweet-tart, 5

Avocados, 2

Bell peppers, green, 1

Bell peppers, red, 3

Bing cherries, frozen, 1½ cups

Broccoli, 1 head

Brussels sprouts, 2 cups

Cabbage, 1 large head, or
1 (14-ounce) bag coleslaw mix

Carrots, 11

Celery, 1 bunch

Chives, 1 bunch

Cilantro, 1 bunch

Fennel bulbs, 2

Garlic, fresh, 2 large heads

Ginger, fresh, 1 (6-inch) piece

Jalapeño peppers, 2

Kale, 1 bunch

Lemon, 1

Limes, 3

Onions, red, 5

Onions, yellow, 2

Oranges, 5

Papaya, 1

Pomegranate, 1, or
pomegranate arils
(seeds), ½ cup

Potato, russet, large, 1

Scallions, 1 bunch

Shallots, 2

Sweet potatoes, large, 2

Zucchini, 1

**Canned Goods and
Pantry Items**

Black beans, low-sodium,
2 (15.5-ounce) cans

Broth, chicken,
low-sodium, ½ cup

Broth, vegetable,
low-sodium, 6 cups

Kidney beans, low-sodium,
1 (15.5-ounce) can

Macaroni, whole-grain,
1 small box

Pineapple chunks,
canned, 1 cup

Tomatoes, no-salt-added,
chopped, 1 (14-ounce) can

White beans, low-sodium,
1 (15.5-ounce) can

Bread crumbs, whole-wheat,
1 canister

Packaged Goods

Dried fruit of choice, 1 cup

Pecans, chopped, ¼ cup

Salmon, wild-caught,
1 (5-ounce) pouch

**Bread and Bread-Like
Products**

Tortillas, whole-wheat, 6

Beef, Pork, Fish, Poultry

Chicken breast, boneless,
skinless, 4 (3-ounce) pieces
plus 6 ounces

Cod, 12 ounces

Ground beef, extra-lean 95%,
9 ounces

Halibut fillets, skin-on,
4 (3-ounce)

Pork chops, thin-cut, 4

Turkey breast, 93% lean
ground, 9 ounces

Turkey breast, whole, bone-in,
skin-on, 1 (4-pound)

Miscellaneous

Tofu, extra firm, 8 ounces

WEEK 3 TIPS

This week is light for meal prep for breakfast and lunch so look ahead at the dinner recipes and gauge if you want to do any prep for those, like chopping onions and peppers for Monday night's stir-fry. I include some leftovers this week for your lunches, so the prep is easy—just divvy them up into storage containers and enjoy the next day!

This week, you'll modify a traditional meat loaf recipe by mixing ground turkey breast with ground beef, reducing its fat calories by 50 percent. I promise, no one will notice the difference!

Looking ahead to Week 3's meal preparation:

On Sunday:

Make a batch of slow-cooker steel-cut oats for Monday and Friday. Or if you have some frozen from Week 1, remove them from the freezer.

Prepare the Asian vinaigrette, which can be kept, refrigerated, for up to 1 week.

Cook 3 ounces of chicken for Monday's lunch.

On Thursday:

Save 3 ounces of cooked chicken (before it is seasoned) from dinner for Friday's lunch.

WEEK 4

You're rounding third base and almost home, and by now you should be feeling pretty good! Eliminating excess sweets and processed food reduces lots of extra calories in your diet, so you may see a difference on the scale or in how your clothes fit. Even though good health is a reward in itself, it's also nice to treat yourself to something special for what you have accomplished. Rewards don't need to be food—get a massage, go to a movie, or just relax and have a fun night out with the family. You have earned it!

WEEK 4 MEAL PLAN

	BREAKFAST	LUNCH	DINNER	SNACKS AND DESSERT
Sunday	Tomato and Spinach Frittata (page 56)	Open-Faced Turkey Burger Caprese (page 73)	Mediterranean Lamb Rib Chops with Roasted Fennel (page 119)	Choose one or two snacks each day from the snack list provided below, and treat yourself to some homemade, yummy desserts this week!
Monday	Spiced Apple Walnut Overnight Oats (page 55)	Minestrone Soup (page 65)	Salmon Cakes with Avocado Salsa (page 122)	Veggie sticks with 2 tablespoons hummus or ¼ cup low-fat yogurt dip
Tuesday	Juicy Cherry Smoothie (page 52)	Salmon and Arugula Salad with Blackberry Vinaigrette (page 70)	Chicken Tacos (page 100)	3 cups unsalted popcorn 1 cup melon chunks, grapes, berries, or cherries
Wednesday	Tomato and Spinach Frittata (leftovers)	Chicken Tacos (leftovers)	Lentil Barley Stew (page 85)	1 small piece of fruit 3 pieces of dried fruit (especially cherries; apricots, prunes, dates)
Thursday	Honeyed Orange Pomegranate Yogurt (page 53)	Spinach, Walnut, and Strawberry Salad with Citrus Vinaigrette (page 68)	Turkey Piccata with Whole-Wheat Penne (page 96)	¾ cup low-fat milk with 2 graham cracker squares 10 unsalted almonds or 2 whole walnuts
Friday	Spiced Apple Walnut Overnight Oats (leftovers)	Lentil Barley Stew (leftovers)	Southwestern Buddha Bowl (page 104)	5 ounces low-fat vanilla Greek or Icelandic-style yogurt 4 whole-grain crackers and 1 ounce low-fat Cheddar or string cheese
Saturday	Red Bell Pepper Omelet (page 60)	Greek Turkey Burger (page 74)	Pork Tenderloin and Greens with Mustard Sauce (page 108)	4 whole-grain crackers with 2 tablespoons hummus or 1 tablespoon all-natural peanut butter

WEEK 4 SHOPPING LIST

Eggs and Dairy

Cheese, feta, ¼ cup

Cheese, shredded Monterey Jack, ¼ cup

Eggs, large, 1½ dozen

Milk, low-fat, 2½ cups

Yogurt, plain low-fat Greek, 1 quart

Produce

Avocados, 3

Baby arugula, 4½ cups

Baby spinach, 6 cups

Bell pepper, red, 2

Blackberries, ½ cup

Bing cherries, frozen, 1½ cups

Carrots, 4

Celery, 1 bunch

Cilantro, 1 bunch

Cucumber, 1

Dill, 1 small bunch

Garlic, 2 heads

Ginger, fresh, 1 (5-inch) piece

Lemons, 3

Limes, 6

Lettuce, 1 head

Parsley, Italian, 1 bunch

Pomegranate, 1, or pomegranate arils (seeds), ½ cup

Onions, red, 2

Onions, yellow, 3

Oranges, 2

Scallions, 1 bunch

Shallots, 4

Strawberries, 1 (1-pound) package

Swiss chard, 1 bunch

Tomatoes, 3

Tomatoes, cherry, 10

Zucchini, 1

Canned Goods and Pantry Items

Barley, pearl, 1 box

Bread crumbs, whole-wheat, 1 container

Broth, low-sodium chicken, 1 cup

Broth, low-sodium vegetable, 2½ quarts

Kidney beans, low-sodium, 1 (15.5-ounce) can

Lentils, dried, 1 package

Oats, old-fashioned, rolled, 1 container

Pasta, macaroni, whole-grain, 1 cup

Pasta, penne, whole-wheat, 4 ounces

Rice, brown, ½ cup uncooked

Tomatoes, low-sodium, crushed, 1 (15.5-ounce) can

Tomatoes, no-salt-added, chopped, 1 (14-ounce) can

Packaged Items

Dried apples, ¼ cup

Salmon, wild-caught, 1 (5-ounce) pouch

Walnuts, chopped, ¾ cup

Bread and Bread-Like Items

Bread, whole-grain, thin-sliced, 1 loaf

Corn tortillas, soft, 8

Hamburger buns, whole-grain, 4

Beef, Pork, Fish, Poultry

Chicken breast, boneless, skinless, 12 ounces

Chicken breast, ground, 12 ounces

Pork tenderloin, 1 (12-ounce)

Salmon, 12 ounces

Turkey breast: cutlets, 4 (3-ounce)

Turkey, 99% extra-lean ground, 12 ounces

Miscellaneous

Bay leaves

Capers, 1 jar

WEEK 4 TIPS

By now, you may be a little low on some of the pantry items like extra-virgin olive oil, apple cider vinegar, nuts, and dried fruits. You should be managing well with the dried spices, as they go a long way. Remember to keep them away from moisture, stored in a dry place like a cabinet versus on top of a stove shelf where steam from cooking can get to them.

Looking ahead to Week 4's meal preparation:

On Sunday:

- Prepare the blackberry vinaigrette for Tuesday's lunch, which can be kept, refrigerated, for up to 3 days.

- Prepare the citrus vinaigrette for Thursday's lunch, which can be kept, refrigerated, for up to 5 days.

- Feel free to swap salad dressings if you prefer one taste over the other. As noted earlier, there is no substitution for taste when it comes to fresh ingredients, and bottled dressings are loaded with salt and sugar.

This week's menu features many DASH-friendly, hearty bean-based meals. According to research studies, purine-containing vegetables and beans do not raise uric acid levels, and may help reduce the risk of gout flares.

Once this week is done, you can continue with the same menu rotation until you feel more comfortable with planning your own meals. There are plenty more recipes in the book that are not included in this 28-day meal plan for you to enjoy, too. I just couldn't fit them all into one month!

BEYOND THE 4 WEEKS

Congratulations! You have just completed the first 28 days of your gout-friendly journey. Not only has the past month paved a path to understanding the fundamentals of healthy eating, but science tells us that incorporating these healthy foods into your daily menu plan can diminish the risk of a gout flare. Your continued commitment to eating well, following your health care provider's medical advice, and taking good care of yourself are key to seeing positive results and living a pain-free life.

HOLIDAYS, BIRTHDAYS, AND SOCIAL EVENTS

In the introduction, I discussed how people with gout can feel socially isolated. It's a lot easier to control your meals when you prepare them yourself, but, realistically, we all have social engagements we want to enjoy. While desserts are always appealing, they can add 500 extra calories to a meal, so limit yourself to a smaller serving. Here are some other tips to help you navigate special occasions:

Be mindful: Mindfulness is the practice of paying close attention to what you are doing or, in this case, eating. Get a sense of when you are really hungry versus how the mood strikes you. Be conscious and in the moment when eating. Listen to your body.

Eat a small meal or snack before the party so you are not hungry when you arrive.

Have a taste of some of the special foods offered, but limit portion sizes. And remember to eat slowly!

Fill your plate with DASH-friendly vegetables.

Stay well hydrated with seltzer water with vitamin C–rich lemon or lime juice.

Focus on enjoying conversations and having a good time rather than eating.

VACATIONS

We all work hard and deserve a vacation, but that doesn't include taking a break from healthy eating. No one wants a vacation ruined with a side trip to the emergency room. One physician I work with noted that he sees more gout attacks in the summer months. A higher intake of seafood and alcohol on vacation with a risk of dehydration can lead to a perfect storm for having a gout attack! So, it's important to maintain a gout-friendly diet even on vacation. Just as you plan ahead for what to wear, decide what you will eat. If you are staying at a spot with cooking facilities, make up a grocery list and menu ideas before you leave home. We've given you a bundle of great-tasting recipes to choose from. Pack plenty of healthy snacks that can fuel all the activities planned and keep you satiated. If you are staying in a hotel, request a room with a microwave and refrigerator so you can store your snacks or leftovers and reheat them the next day. Refer also to the following restaurant tips.

RESTAURANTS

Did you know going out to dinner can cost you up to 1,500 calories—from appetizer to dessert? It's nice not to have to cook some nights, but don't sabotage all your efforts in one night. Have a plan and be prepared before you walk through the restaurant's door.

Start by going online and viewing the menu before you visit a restaurant. Ask your server specific questions regarding the meal preparation and ingredients; they are well trained to accommodate questions and special requests. Have a light snack if dinner is going to be late; arriving at a restaurant in a starved state can lead to ordering the wrong foods and eating too much. Eat small amounts and moderate your alcohol intake. A good way to limit sodium and calories is to share your meal or eat half of it at the restaurant and take the rest home.

Strategies for Dining Out

TYPE OF FOOD	AVOID OR LIMIT	BETTER CHOICES
Buffet	Limit red meats and seafood (shrimp, lobster, sardines) to a 6-ounce serving	Grilled, sautéed, or broiled fish or chicken
	Soups (high in sodium); olives; pickles; bacon bits; salted nuts; croutons; olive salads; macaroni salad; relishes; pickles	Roasted, steamed, or grilled vegetables
	No entrées or vegetables in creamed or cheese sauces (escalloped, au gratin)	Salad bar; coleslaw; gelatin salads; cottage cheese; oil-and-vinegar or vinaigrette dressing
	No fried foods	
	No marinated meats	
	No creamy salad dressings or sour cream	
Asian	No fried foods or spareribs	Steamed entrées, vegetables, tofu
	Fried egg rolls; Peking ravioli; dim sum; pot stickers; soy sauce; teriyaki sauce	Rice (brown preferred), plain noodles; lettuce roll-ups
		Request that your food be prepared without soy sauce, fish sauce, or MSG; all are high in sodium
Italian	Alfredo, Bolognese, or carbonara sauce	Marinara (can be high in sodium, so watch amount); pesto; piccata (capers can add sodium)
	Small portion (less than 6 ounces) of clam or mussel dishes	Plain pasta (e.g., spaghetti, fettuccini, penne, tortellini, ravioli)
	Use grated cheese in moderation	Breadsticks; bread with extra-virgin olive oil
	Buttered garlic bread	Wine sauces (e.g., marsala)
	Creamy salad dressings	Mixed-greens salad with oil-and-vinegar or vinaigrette dressing

TYPE OF FOOD	AVOID OR LIMIT	BETTER CHOICES
Mexican	Sour cream Fried entrées or sides Green chili (if cream-based) Fried taco shells Limit red meat to 6-ounce servings (e.g., enchiladas filled with minced meat) Watch amount of cheese	Baked, broiled, grilled, or steamed chicken or fish dishes preferred Plain rice (brown preferred); soft tacos, burritos, fajitas Salsa (no cream) Avocado; guacamole
Mediterranean	Spinach-filled phyllo pastries, sausage rolls, falafel, scalloped potatoes; risotto (high sodium if chicken broth is not homemade); creamed sauces Limit kebab/skewered lean meats and seafood (shrimp, lobster) to 6 ounces Feta cheese is higher in sodium, so limit amount eaten	Grilled, sautéed, or broiled fish or chicken Wine sauces Roasted, steamed, or grilled vegetables; rice; potato; couscous; tabbouleh Mixed-greens salad with oil-and-vinegar or vinaigrette dressing
Barbecue	Barbecue sauce, steak sauce, horseradish, sausage, hot dogs, corn bread; MSG or teriyaki sauce Limit red meats (grilled or broiled) and seafood (shrimp, lobster) to 6 ounces; pulled meats (pork, beef, and chicken) are high in sodium, so consider sharing a meal	Grilled or broiled chicken or fish; 2-inch square of corn bread; grilled vegetables Marinades with wine, lemon juice, oil, vinegar, garlic, honey, herbs, and spices
Dessert	Dough piecrusts; milk chocolate; coconut; cheesecake; custard; puddings; ice cream; gelato	All fresh fruit or canned, unsweetened fruit; sugar cookies, angel food cake; gelatin; low-fat frozen yogurt or light ice cream; puddings with low-fat milk; graham crackers; cobblers or crisps; graham cracker piecrusts; dark chocolate square

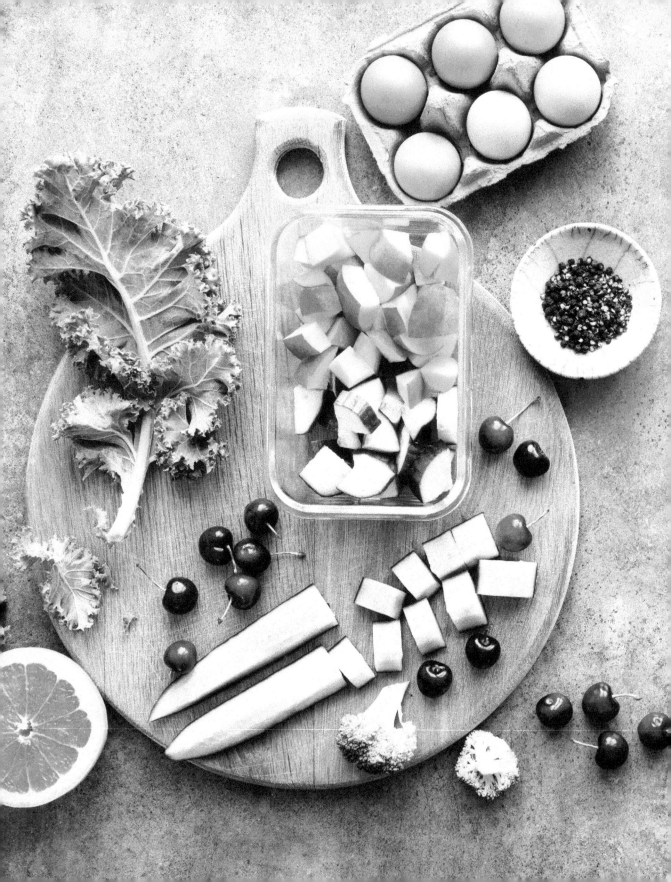

PART TWO

The Recipes

The recipes that follow are not only designed to be gout friendly, they have also been developed to support heart and kidney health. They are packed with nutrient-dense foods as prescribed in the DASH diet, including the fruits, vegetables, whole grains, legumes, and lean protein that are so good for you. The recipes are also marked as Gluten Free, Kidney Friendly, Diabetes Friendly, and Vegan or Vegetarian to help you identify whether the ingredients are permitted within the scope of your personal dietary needs or preferences. I hope you enjoy some new tastes and flavors!

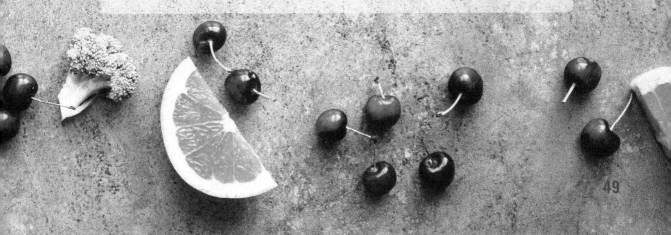

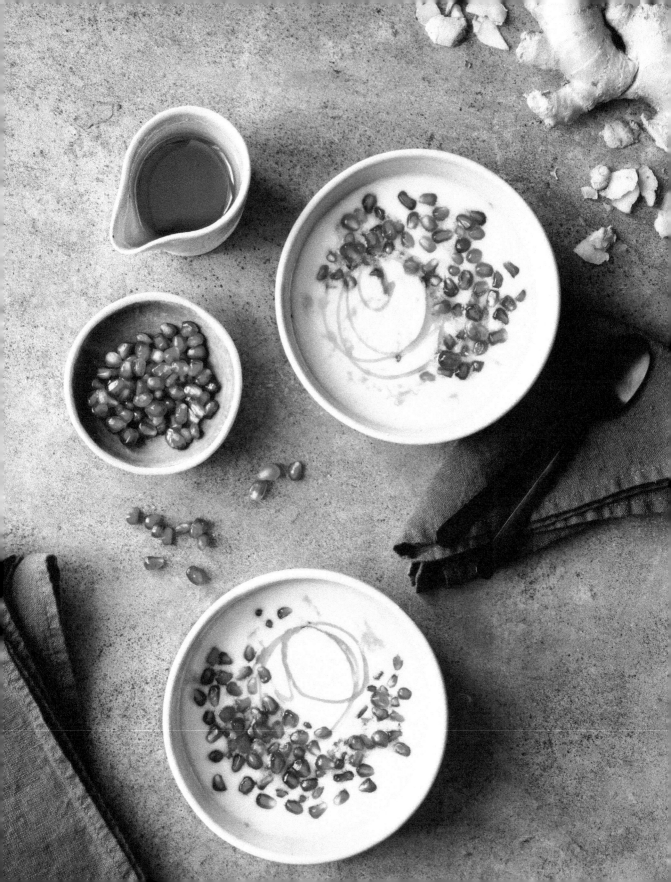

CHAPTER 4

Juicy Cherry Smoothie

SERVES 2   PREP TIME: 5 MINUTES

DIABETES FRIENDLY • GLUTEN FREE • KIDNEY FRIENDLY • VEGAN OPTION • VEGETARIAN

Smoothies make a great breakfast for weekdays because they are quick and easy. Just toss the ingredients into a blender and you're good to go. You can also keep leftovers in the fridge for about 3 days and just reblend before serving.

2 cups low-fat milk or nondairy milk, such as unsweetened almond milk or soy milk, for a vegan smoothie

1½ cups frozen pitted bing cherries

1 tablespoon chia seeds

½ teaspoon grated peeled fresh ginger or turmeric (optional)

½ cup crushed ice

PER SERVING (2 CUPS)
Total Calories: 220; Total Fat: 4g; Saturated Fat: 1g;
Cholesterol: 10mg; Sodium: 130mg;
Potassium: 71mg; Total Carbohydrate: 33g;
Fiber: 5g; Sugars: 26g; Protein: 11g

In a blender, combine the milk, cherries, chia seeds, ginger (if using), and ice. Blend until smooth.

VARIATION TIP: Smoothies are extremely customizable. Replace the cherries with 1½ cups of any type of chopped soft fruit, such as peaches or berries. The ginger, or turmeric, adds anti-inflammatory power. If you prefer a slightly sweeter smoothie, add 1 tablespoon honey or 1 packet of stevia.

Honeyed Orange Pomegranate Yogurt

SERVES 1   PREP TIME: 5 MINUTES

GLUTEN FREE • KIDNEY FRIENDLY • VEGETARIAN

Yogurt makes a good moderate-protein snack or breakfast choice. Greek yogurt has more protein than regular yogurt, so it's a good add-in. Because this is so quick and easy, you can make a single serving at a time. It's helpful to have a manual citrus juicer, but you can also squeeze the juice from the oranges using just your hands. To zest the orange, use a rasp-style grater and make sure you don't get any of the pith (white part), which is bitter.

1 cup plain low-fat Greek yogurt

Zest of ½ orange

Juice of ½ orange

1 tablespoon honey

½ teaspoon grated fresh ginger or turmeric (optional)

½ cup pomegranate seeds (arils; see ingredient tip)

PER SERVING (1 CUP)
Total Calories: 328; Total Fat: 6g; Saturated Fat: 3g; Cholesterol: 35mg; Sodium: 144mg; Potassium: 69mg; Total Carbohydrate: 49g; Fiber: 3g; Sugars: 36g; Protein: 23g

1. In a small bowl, stir together the yogurt, orange zest and juice, honey, and ginger (if using).

2. Serve with the pomegranate seeds sprinkled over the top.

VARIATION TIP: This is easy to customize to your taste. Omit the juice and just stir in the honey. Add up to ½ cup of any chopped soft fruit you like.

INGREDIENT TIP: If you can't find pomegranate seeds already out of their shell, you can extract the seeds by halving the pomegranate, holding the fruit cut-side down over a plate or bowl, and firmly tapping the shell with a wooden spoon.

Slow-Cooker Fruit 'n' Oats

SERVES 6   PREP TIME: 5 MINUTES   COOK TIME: 6 HOURS, 30 MINUTES

GLUTEN FREE OPTION • **KIDNEY FRIENDLY** • VEGAN OPTION

Not all oats are gluten free because they can be cross-contaminated during processing. So, if you need them to be, make sure you purchase a brand that is certified gluten free. Make this recipe while you sleep and keep handy leftovers in the fridge for up to 5 days. Reheat in the microwave.

1 cup steel-cut oats (see ingredient tip)

4 cups water

½ cup freshly squeezed orange juice, or more water

Zest of ½ orange

¼ cup chia seeds

1 cup dried unsweetened fruit, such as apples, cranberries, raisins, etc.

¼ cup honey, or pure maple syrup for a vegan option

1 teaspoon grated peeled fresh ginger

1 teaspoon ground cinnamon

¼ cup chopped pecans (optional)

1. In a slow cooker, stir together the oats, water, orange juice, orange zest, chia seeds, dried fruit, honey, ginger, and cinnamon.

2. Cover the cooker and set to low heat. Cook for 6 to 8 hours.

3. Stir in the nuts (if using) before serving.

INGREDIENT TIP: Don't use rolled oats, as they won't hold up in a slow cooker. You must use the heartier steel-cut oats for this recipe.

PER SERVING (1 CUP) USING DRIED UNSWEETENED CRANBERRIES
Total Calories: 259; Total Fat: 4g; Saturated Fat: 0g; Cholesterol: 0mg; Sodium: 1mg; Potassium: 88mg; Total Carbohydrate: 52g; Fiber: 7g; Sugars: 27g; Protein: 6g

Spiced Apple Walnut Overnight Oats

SERVES 1   **PREP TIME: 5 MINUTES**   **COOK TIME: OVERNIGHT RESTING**

DIABETES FRIENDLY • KIDNEY FRIENDLY • VEGAN OPTION • VEGETARIAN

This is a good breakfast if you just need to grab and go in the morning. It's served chilled, so there's no need to heat it, and it uses old-fashioned oats. Don't use instant oats, which are too mushy. It's also easy to customize to suit your preferences.

½ cup low-fat milk, or nondairy unsweetened milk such as almond or rice milk, for a vegan option

¼ cup plain low-fat Greek yogurt (omit for vegan oats)

½ cup old-fashioned rolled oats

¼ cup dried apples

2 tablespoons chopped walnuts

2 teaspoons chia seeds

½ teaspoon ground cinnamon

1 tablespoon pure maple syrup (optional)

PER SERVING (1½ CUPS)
Total Calories: 430; Total Fat: 17g; Saturated Fat: 3g; Cholesterol: 16mg; Sodium: 114mg; Potassium: 134mg; Total Carbohydrate: 55g; Fiber: 10g; Sugars: 20g; Protein: 18g

1. In a small mason jar, combine the milk, yogurt, oats, dried apples, walnuts, chia seeds, and cinnamon. Mix well. Cover and refrigerate for at least 5 hours, or overnight.

2. If needed in the morning, stir in a little more liquid to thin to your desired consistency. If you don't prefer cold oats, heat them in the microwave for 1 to 2 minutes on high power. Drizzle maple syrup on top, if desired.

VARIATION TIP: Add ¼ cup of any dried or fresh fruit you want in place of the apples. If using fresh fruit, stir it in just before serving. You can also switch spices—try pumpkin pie spice, ginger, or nutmeg for a different flavor profile. Try topping it with nut butter, or stir in some pumpkin purée before eating.

Tomato and Spinach Frittata

SERVES 2 PREP TIME: 10 MINUTES COOK TIME: 15 MINUTES

DIABETES FRIENDLY • GLUTEN FREE • KIDNEY FRIENDLY

Frittatas are a quick breakfast, even on busy mornings. They also keep well, so you can refrigerate extra servings for up to 3 days and reheat in the microwave for about 1 minute on high power. Served with a side salad, this also makes a great lunch or light dinner.

1 tablespoon extra-virgin olive oil

½ onion, thinly sliced

2 cups fresh baby spinach

2 large eggs (see ingredient tip)

4 large egg whites

¼ teaspoon freshly ground black pepper

10 cherry tomatoes, halved

3 tablespoons grated Parmesan cheese

PER SERVING (½ FRITTATA)
Total Calories: 233; Total Fat: 15g;
Saturated Fat: 4.5g; Cholesterol: 219mg;
Sodium: 351mg; Potassium: 340mg;
Total Carbohydrate: 8g; Fiber: 2g;
Sugars: 2g; Protein: 18g

1. Preheat the broiler to high and adjust a rack to the top position.

2. In a 10-inch ovenproof nonstick skillet over medium-high heat, heat the olive oil until it shimmers.

3. Add the onion and cook for 5 minutes, stirring occasionally. Add the spinach and cook for 1 minute more, stirring occasionally. Spread the vegetables in an even layer on the bottom of the skillet and reduce the heat to medium.

4. In a small bowl, whisk the eggs, egg whites, and pepper. Carefully pour the eggs over the vegetables. Cook, without stirring, until the eggs set around the edges of the pan. Use a spatula to pull the set eggs away from the edges of the pan and tilt the pan so uncooked egg flows underneath. Cook for 1 to 2 minutes more until the eggs set. Remove from the heat.

5. Arrange the tomatoes on top of the eggs and sprinkle with the cheese. Place the skillet under the broiler for about 5 minutes until the eggs set and the cheese melts.

VARIATION TIP: Frittatas are easy to customize. Replace the onion with ½ bell pepper, sliced, or replace the spinach with chopped, stemmed kale or Swiss chard, or a small chopped zucchini.

INGREDIENT TIP: If you purchase egg whites, 3 tablespoons equals 1 egg white.

Black Bean Breakfast Burrito

SERVES 4   PREP TIME: 10 MINUTES   COOK TIME: 20 MINUTES

DIABETES FRIENDLY • KIDNEY FRIENDLY • VEGETARIAN

Breakfast burritos are portable and reheatable, so you can make them ahead and take them with you. Reheat in the microwave wrapped in a damp paper towel for 1 to 2 minutes on high power. These burritos keep, refrigerated, for up to 5 days. You can also double the recipe and freeze them for up to 6 months.

1 tablespoon extra-virgin olive oil

6 scallions, white and green parts, finely chopped

1 jalapeño pepper, seeded and chopped

1 (15.5-ounce) can low-sodium black beans, drained and rinsed

2 large eggs

4 large egg whites

½ teaspoon ground cumin

½ teaspoon chili powder

½ teaspoon garlic powder

4 (8-inch) whole-wheat tortillas

½ cup shredded low-fat Cheddar cheese

½ avocado, finely chopped

¼ cup chopped fresh cilantro

1. Preheat the oven to 350°F. Line a rimmed baking sheet with parchment paper. Set aside.

2. In a large nonstick skillet over medium-high heat, heat the olive oil until it shimmers.

3. Add the scallions and jalapeño. Cook for about 4 minutes, stirring occasionally, until the vegetables are soft.

4. Add the black beans. Cook for 1 minute, stirring. Reduce the heat to medium.

PER SERVING (1 BURRITO)
Total Calories: 375; Total Fat: 14g;
Saturated Fat: 4g; Cholesterol: 111mg;
Sodium: 397mg; Potassium: 243mg;
Total Carbohydrate: 43g; Fiber: 10g;
Sugars: 3g; Protein: 20g

5. In a small bowl, whisk the eggs, egg whites, cumin, chili powder, and garlic powder. Add the eggs to the skillet. Cook for 3 to 4 minutes, scrambling the eggs, until set.

6. Spoon the mixture onto the tortillas and top with the cheese. Roll into a burrito and place on the prepared baking sheet. Bake for about 10 minutes until heated through.

7. Serve topped with avocado and cilantro.

VARIATION TIP: It's easy to increase the veggies in your burrito. Just add up to 1 cup chopped veggies, such as bell pepper or broccoli, when you cook the onions and jalapeño.

Red Bell Pepper Omelet

SERVES 2   PREP TIME: 10 MINUTES   COOK TIME: 15 MINUTES

DIABETES FRIENDLY • GLUTEN FREE • KIDNEY FRIENDLY • VEGETARIAN

Like frittatas and scrambled eggs, omelets are also easy to customize to satisfy your tastes and add variety to your meals. This version has red bell peppers, which are high in vitamin C and have a nice sweet flavor. You can refrigerate leftovers for up to 5 days and reheat in the microwave for about 1 minute on high power.

1 tablespoon extra-virgin olive oil

1 red bell pepper, seeded and sliced

1 garlic clove, minced

2 large eggs

4 large egg whites

¼ teaspoon freshly ground black pepper

¼ teaspoon sea salt

¼ cup shredded Monterey Jack cheese

PER SERVING (½ OMELET)
Total Calories: 232; Total Fat: 16g;
Saturated Fat: 5g; Cholesterol: 226mg;
Sodium: 556mg; Potassium: 219mg;
Total Carbohydrate: 5g; Fiber: 1g;
Sugars: 0g; Protein: 17g

1. In a 10-inch nonstick skillet over medium-high heat, heat the olive oil until it shimmers.

2. Add the bell pepper. Cook for about 5 minutes, stirring occasionally, until soft.

3. Add the garlic and cook for 30 seconds, stirring constantly. Arrange the red bell peppers in the bottom of the skillet in a single layer. Reduce the heat to medium.

4. In a small bowl, whisk the eggs, egg whites, pepper, and salt. Pour the eggs over the red bell peppers. Cook, without stirring, allowing the eggs to set around the edges. Using a spatula, pull the edges away from the sides of the pan, tilt the pan, and allow the uncooked eggs to flow underneath. Cook for about 4 minutes more until the eggs set.

5. Sprinkle the cheese over the eggs. Turn off the heat. Using a spatula, fold the omelet in half and cover. Let sit, covered, until the cheese melts, about 1 minute.

Salmon and Kale Scramble

SERVES 4 PREP TIME: 10 MINUTES COOK TIME: 15 MINUTES

DIABETES FRIENDLY • GLUTEN FREE • KIDNEY FRIENDLY

Loaded with anti-inflammatory heart-healthy omega-3 fatty acids from the salmon, this is a delicious and quick breakfast. For simplicity, use wild-caught salmon in a pouch, or you can also use fresh poached salmon if you prefer.

1 tablespoon extra-virgin olive oil

1 shallot, minced

2 cups chopped stemmed kale

1 (5-ounce) pouch wild-caught salmon

2 large eggs

6 large egg whites

¼ teaspoon freshly ground black pepper

1 teaspoon dried dill

PER SERVING (1½ CUPS)
Total Calories: 141; Total Fat: 7g; Saturated Fat: 2g;
Cholesterol: 118mg; Sodium: 302mg;
Potassium: 98mg; Total Carbohydrate: 3g;
Fiber: 0g; Sugars: 0g; Protein: 15g

1. In a 12-inch nonstick skillet over medium-high heat, heat the olive oil until it shimmers.

2. Add the shallot and kale. Cook for about 7 minutes, stirring occasionally, until the vegetables are soft.

3. Add the salmon. Cook, stirring, for 1 minute more. Reduce the heat to medium.

4. In a small bowl, whisk the egg yolks, egg whites, pepper, and dill. Add the eggs to the vegetables. Cook for about 4 minutes, stirring occasionally, until the eggs are set.

VARIATION TIP: You can add all sorts of ingredients to your scrambled eggs to add variety. Replace the salmon with 5 ounces of another low-sodium, low-fat meat, such as ground turkey sausage, and replace the kale with vegetables like chopped asparagus (2 cups) or chopped bell pepper.

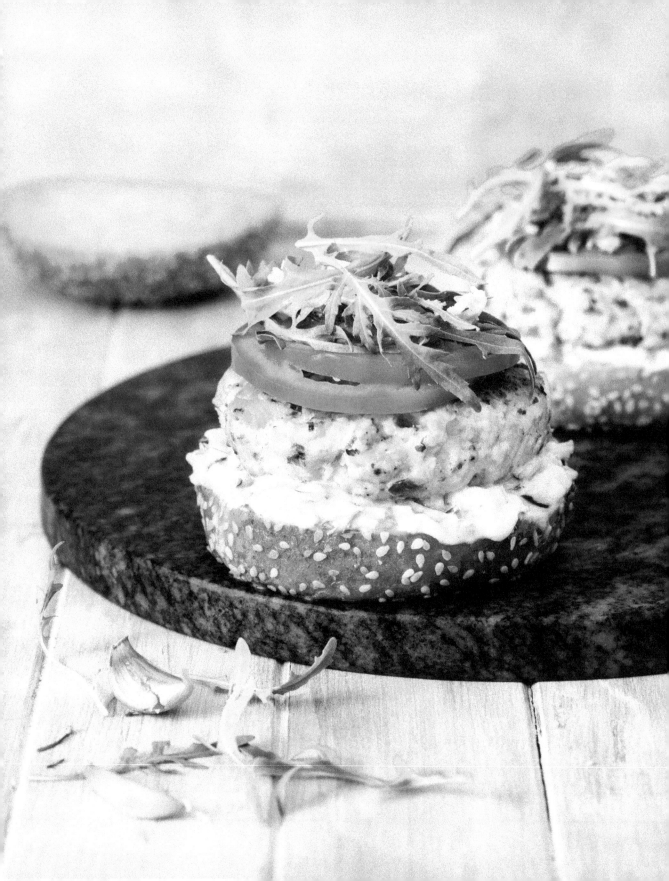

CHAPTER 5

Tuscan Bean, Kale, and Turkey Sausage Soup

SERVES 4   PREP TIME: 10 MINUTES   COOK TIME: 25 MINUTES

DIABETES FRIENDLY • KIDNEY FRIENDLY

This hearty soup freezes and travels well, so mix up a double batch and save it in single-serving containers for easy meals in a snap. Reheat on the stove top or in the microwave. It will keep, refrigerated, for up to 5 days. This is a fragrant, flavorful soup the whole family will enjoy.

1 tablespoon extra-virgin olive oil

8 ounces Italian turkey sausage (see ingredient tip)

1 onion, chopped

1 red bell pepper, seeded and chopped

2 cups chopped stemmed kale

6 garlic cloves, minced

1 (15.5-ounce) can low-sodium white beans (such as cannellini), drained and rinsed

1 teaspoon dried Italian seasoning

1 (14-ounce) can no-salt-added diced tomatoes, undrained

4 cups low-sodium chicken broth, or Poultry Broth (page 148)

¼ teaspoon freshly ground black pepper

Pinch red pepper flakes (optional)

1. In a large pot over medium-high heat, heat the olive oil until it shimmers.
2. Add the turkey sausage and cook for about 5 minutes, stirring and crumbling with a spoon, until browned.
3. Add the onion, red bell pepper, and kale. Cook for 5 minutes, stirring.
4. Add the garlic and cook for 30 seconds, stirring constantly.
5. Add the white beans, Italian seasoning, tomatoes and their juice, chicken broth, black pepper, and red pepper flakes (if using). Bring to a simmer and reduce the heat to medium-low. Cook for 5 minutes more, stirring occasionally.

INGREDIENT TIP: If the sausage comes in casings, score the casing with a sharp knife and remove the meat from it to make a bulk sausage that cooks and crumbles easily.

PER SERVING (2 CUPS)
Total Calories: 254; Total Fat: 6g; Saturated Fat: 1g; Cholesterol: 23mg; Sodium: 463mg; Potassium: 392mg; Total Carbohydrate: 29g; Fiber: 7g; Sugars: 6g; Protein: 21g

Minestrone Soup

SERVES 4   PREP TIME: 10 MINUTES   COOK TIME: 20 MINUTES

DIABETES FRIENDLY • VEGAN

Eating minestrone is a flavorful way to get your veggies. While meatless, the soup is hearty, fragrant, and rich. You can make a double batch and freeze individual 2-cup portions for up to 6 months. Enjoy this soup alone or with a half sandwich or simple salad for a heartier meal.

2 tablespoons extra-virgin olive oil

1 onion, chopped

1 red bell pepper, seeded and chopped

2 carrots, chopped

1 celery stalk, chopped

1 medium zucchini, chopped

6 garlic cloves, minced

1 (14-ounce) can no-salt-added chopped tomatoes, undrained

1 teaspoon dried Italian seasoning

¼ teaspoon freshly ground black pepper

4 cups low-sodium vegetable broth

1 cup whole-grain macaroni

1 cup canned low-sodium kidney beans, drained and rinsed

Pinch red pepper flakes

PER SERVING (2 CUPS)
Total Calories: 244; Total Fat: 7g; Saturated Fat: 1g; Cholesterol: 0mg; Sodium: 121mg; Potassium: 665mg; Total Carbohydrate: 37g; Fiber: 8g; Sugars: 7g; Protein: 10g

1. In a large pot over medium-high heat, heat the olive oil until it shimmers. Add the onion, red bell pepper, carrots, celery, and zucchini. Cook for about 5 minutes, stirring, until the vegetables begin to soften.

2. Add the garlic and cook for 30 seconds, stirring constantly.

3. Stir in the tomatoes and their juice, Italian seasoning, black pepper, and vegetable broth. Bring the soup to a simmer.

4. Stir in the macaroni, kidney beans, and red pepper flakes. Bring to a boil. Cook for about 8 minutes, stirring occasionally, until the pasta is al dente.

VARIATION TIP: Any seasonal vegetable works in this soup. Consider adding up to 1 cup green beans, chopped winter squash, or fresh peas.

Chicken Zoodle Soup with White Beans

SERVES 4   PREP TIME: 10 MINUTES   COOK TIME: 20 MINUTES

DIABETES FRIENDLY • GLUTEN FREE • KIDNEY FRIENDLY

If your grocery store carries raw chicken tenders, which are trimmed from whole chicken breasts, they are easiest to use for this recipe. If you can't find them, use sliced fresh chicken breast instead. To make zucchini noodles, use a spiralizer or vegetable peeler to peel the zucchini in long, wide strips down the length of the zucchini.

2 tablespoons extra-virgin olive oil

1 onion, chopped

8 ounces boneless, skinless chicken tenders, cut into 1-inch pieces

1 carrot, chopped

1 celery stalk, chopped

4 garlic cloves, minced

5 cups low-sodium chicken broth or Poultry Broth (page 148)

2 teaspoons dried rosemary

Juice of 1 lemon

¼ teaspoon sea salt

¼ teaspoon freshly ground black pepper

1 (15.5-ounce) can low-sodium white beans, drained and rinsed

2 zucchini, unpeeled, cut into wide noodles (see headnote and ingredient tip)

1. In a large pot over medium-high heat, heat the olive oil until it shimmers. Add the onion and chicken. Cook for about 5 minutes, stirring occasionally, until opaque.

2. Add the carrot and celery. Cook for about 5 minutes more, stirring, until the vegetables begin to soften.

3. Add the garlic. Cook for 30 seconds, stirring constantly.

PER SERVING (2 CUPS)
Total Calories: 274; Total Fat: 9g;
Saturated Fat: 2g; Cholesterol: 32mg;
Sodium: 281mg; Potassium: 398mg;
Total Carbohydrate: 27g; Fiber: 7g;
Sugars: 5g; Protein: 22g

4. Stir in the chicken broth, rosemary, lemon juice, salt, and pepper. Bring to a simmer.

5. Add the beans and zucchini noodles. Cook for 5 minutes, stirring.

INGREDIENT TIP: Don't want to mess with making zucchini noodles? Look for spiralized zucchini in your grocery store's produce aisle or use 2 ounces whole-grain egg noodles instead, or 1 cup cooked brown rice to keep it gluten free.

Spinach, Walnut, and Strawberry Salad with Citrus Vinaigrette

SERVES 2   PREP TIME: 10 MINUTES

DIABETES FRIENDLY • GLUTEN FREE • **KIDNEY FRIENDLY** • VEGAN

With a citrusy dressing and crunchy walnuts, this salad makes a great light lunch, snack, or side for a main course. Using baby spinach keeps the greens bite-size and tender, and saves time in prep because you don't have to tear up the spinach. Both spinach and strawberries are anti-inflammatory and excellent sources of vitamin C.

4 cups fresh baby spinach

2 cups sliced fresh strawberries

½ cup chopped walnuts

¼ cup Citrus Vinaigrette (page 149)

In a large bowl, combine the spinach, strawberries, walnuts, and vinaigrette. Toss to mix.

PER SERVING (ABOUT 3 CUPS)
Total Calories: 341; Total Fat: 27g; Saturated Fat: 3g; Cholesterol: 0mg; Sodium: 197mg; Potassium: 385mg; Total Carbohydrate: 25g; Fiber: 7g; Sugars: 16g; Protein: 7g

PREPARATION TIP: If storing this salad or taking it with you, keep the salad and vinaigrette separate and mix just before eating or the spinach will become soggy. You can also omit the vinaigrette and season this salad simply with 1 tablespoon each of extra-virgin olive oil and vinegar.

Asian Apple and Cabbage Slaw with Roasted Chicken

SERVES 2   PREP TIME: 10 MINUTES

DIABETES FRIENDLY • GLUTEN FREE • KIDNEY FRIENDLY

Using a rotisserie chicken from the grocery store makes this a quick and easy meal, although you can also cook your own skinless chicken breast. If making ahead, keep the slaw and dressing separate and mix it all together just before serving.

1 apple, peeled, cored, and julienned

3 cups shredded green cabbage, or bagged coleslaw mix

4 ounces cooked skinless chicken breast

2 scallions, white and green parts, finely chopped

1 tablespoon sesame seeds, toasted

¼ cup Asian Vinaigrette (page 150)

PER SERVING (ABOUT 2 CUPS)
Total Calories: 236; Total Fat: 10g;
Saturated Fat: 2g; Cholesterol: 32mg;
Sodium: 258mg; Potassium: 521mg;
Total Carbohydrate: 27g; Fiber: 5g;
Sugars: 20g; Protein: 14g

In a large bowl, combine the apple, cabbage, chicken, scallions, sesame seeds, and vinaigrette. Toss to mix.

PREPARATION TIP: To save time peeling and coring apples, use an apple peeler-corer. This is great to have if you work with apples a lot, and it provides thin, even slices you can easily cut into smaller pieces.

Salmon and Arugula Salad with Blackberry Vinaigrette

SERVES 2 PREP TIME: 10 MINUTES

DIABETES FRIENDLY • GLUTEN FREE • KIDNEY FRIENDLY

To make this salad, use either fresh wild-caught salmon you've grilled for about five minutes on an indoor or outdoor grill (to your desired doneness) or precooked wild-caught salmon in a pouch. Either way, this salad is packed with heart-healthy omega-3 fatty acids and anti-inflammatory greens and dark berries.

4 cups baby arugula

5 ounces cooked wild-caught salmon, flaked

2 scallions, white and green parts, finely chopped

¼ cup Blackberry Vinaigrette (page 151)

In a large bowl, combine the arugula, salmon, scallions, and vinaigrette. Toss to mix.

INGREDIENT TIP: This is a good salad to use up any leftover cooked fish, including whitefish, shellfish such as shrimp, or salmon. You can also use chicken or turkey.

PER SERVING (ABOUT 2 CUPS)
Total Calories: 234; Total Fat: 12g;
Saturated Fat: 2g; Cholesterol: 50mg;
Sodium: 192mg; Potassium: 41mg;
Total Carbohydrate: 11g; Fiber: 1g;
Sugars: 9g; Protein: 21g

Chopped Italian Salad

SERVES 4   PREP TIME: 10 MINUTES

DIABETES FRIENDLY • GLUTEN FREE • KIDNEY FRIENDLY

This chopped salad is hearty and travels well. It's also easy to change it up to meet your taste preferences. Include lots of fresh chopped veggies to keep it nutritious and limit any meat you substitute to low-salt versions with a maximum of 3 ounces per serving.

1 cup chopped cooked boneless, skinless chicken breast

3 ounces Canadian bacon, chopped

2 cups cherry tomatoes, halved

1 (14-ounce can) no-salt-added artichoke bottoms, halved

2 ounces shredded mozzarella cheese (about ½ cup)

1 cucumber, chopped

¼ cup fresh basil leaves, torn

¼ cup pine nuts

¼ cup plain low-fat Greek yogurt

¼ cup apple cider vinegar

1 garlic clove, minced

½ teaspoon freshly ground black pepper

1. In a large bowl, combine the chicken, Canadian bacon, tomatoes, artichokes, cheese, cucumber, basil, and pine nuts.

2. In a small bowl, whisk the yogurt, vinegar, garlic, and pepper.

3. Add the dressing to the chicken and vegetables. Toss to combine.

PREPARATION TIP: Lower the total salt content by omitting the Canadian bacon and adding 3 more ounces of chopped cooked chicken.

PER SERVING (1 CUP)
Total Calories: 254; Total Fat: 12g;
Saturated Fat: 3g; Cholesterol: 50mg;
Sodium: 590mg; Potassium: 349mg;
Total Carbohydrate: 14g; Fiber: 5g;
Sugars: 2g; Protein: 24g

Buffalo Chicken Wrap

SERVES 2   PREP TIME: 10 MINUTES   COOK TIME: 10 MINUTES

DIABETES FRIENDLY • KIDNEY FRIENDLY

Wraps are easy to pack for to-go lunches and help you stay on track. You can enjoy this version warm or cold. If you're not a fan of blue cheese, omit it from the slaw. The traditional sauce for buffalo chicken is made with Frank's RedHot, but any Louisiana hot sauce will do. It is also typically made with butter, but we've swapped in olive oil to make this heart healthier.

2 tablespoons extra-virgin olive oil

6 ounces boneless, skinless chicken breast, cut into ½-inch pieces

1 tablespoon Frank's RedHot, or any Louisiana hot sauce

3 carrots, grated

2 tablespoons crumbled blue cheese

¼ cup plain low-fat Greek yogurt

2 scallions, white and green parts, thinly sliced

2 (8-inch) whole-wheat tortillas

PER SERVING (1 WRAP)
Total Calories: 440; Total Fat: 22g;
Saturated Fat: 5g; Cholesterol: 58mg;
Sodium: 603mg; Potassium: 341mg;
Total Carbohydrate: 35g; Fiber: 6g;
Sugars: 7g; Protein: 29g

1. In a large nonstick skillet over medium-high heat, heat the olive oil until it shimmers.

2. Add the chicken. Cook for 5 to 7 minutes, stirring occasionally, until opaque.

3. Add the hot sauce. Cook, stirring, until the meat is coated. Set aside to cool completely.

4. In a medium bowl, stir together the carrots, blue cheese, yogurt, and scallions.

5. Spoon the cooled chicken onto the tortillas. Top with the carrot mixture and wrap.

PREPARATION TIP: Make this more quickly and easily using precooked rotisserie chicken breast from the grocery store with the skin removed. In a medium bowl, combine the chicken, hot sauce, and 1 tablespoon olive oil. No need to cook.

Open-Faced Turkey Burger Caprese

SERVES 4 PREP TIME: 10 MINUTES COOK TIME: 10 MINUTES

DIABETES FRIENDLY • KIDNEY FRIENDLY

With traditional Italian flavors, this dish is especially good when tomatoes and/
or fresh basil are in season. If they are, opt for a juicy heirloom tomato that will
make this burger's flavors really pop.

12 ounces 93% lean ground turkey

1 tablespoon extra-virgin olive oil

½ cup shredded mozzarella cheese

½ cup plain low-fat Greek yogurt

¼ cup fresh basil leaves

1 garlic clove

1 large tomato, chopped

4 slices whole-grain bread, thin-sliced

PER SERVING (1 BURGER)
Total Calories: 304; Total Fat: 14g;
Saturated Fat: 4g; Cholesterol: 72mg;
Sodium: 357mg; Potassium: 116mg;
Total Carbohydrate: 18g; Fiber: 3g;
Sugars: 3g; Protein: 26g

1. Form the ground turkey into 4 patties.

2. In a large nonstick skillet or grill pan
   over medium-high heat, heat the olive oil
   until it shimmers. Add the patties. Cook
   until browned on both sides and cooked
   through, about 7 minutes total.

3. Sprinkle each burger with 2 tablespoons
   of cheese. Turn off the heat, cover the
   skillet, and let sit until the cheese melts.

4. As the turkey cooks, in a blender or
   food processor, combine the yogurt,
   basil, and garlic. Blend until smooth.
   Stir in the chopped tomato. Toast the
   bread, if desired.

5. Serve the burgers on the bread with the
   basil and tomato mixture spooned over
   the top.

INGREDIENT TIP: Try these using 95%
extra-lean ground beef or ground chicken
instead of the turkey.

Greek Turkey Burger

SERVES 4   PREP TIME: 10 MINUTES   COOK TIME: 10 MINUTES

DIABETES FRIENDLY • KIDNEY FRIENDLY

If you're a fan of Mediterranean flavors, you'll love this tasty turkey burger with feta cheese and spinach. It's the perfect meal for a summertime barbecue, and, if you store the bun, condiments, and burger separately, you can make it ahead, reheat the patty in the microwave, and assemble it just before it's time to eat. The cooked burger will keep in the fridge for 3 to 4 days.

12 ounces extra-lean (99%) ground turkey breast

3 garlic cloves, minced, divided

½ red onion, grated and wrung out in a tea towel (see preparation tip)

1 cup fresh baby spinach, chopped

2 tablespoons chopped fresh Italian parsley

1 teaspoon ground cumin

1 teaspoon dried oregano

⅛ teaspoon sea salt

¼ teaspoon freshly ground black pepper

2 tablespoons extra-virgin olive oil

¼ cup feta cheese, crumbled

½ cucumber, minced

1 tablespoon chopped fresh dill

1 tablespoon freshly squeezed lemon juice

½ cup plain low-fat Greek yogurt

4 whole-grain hamburger buns, toasted

4 slices tomato

½ cup arugula

PER SERVING (1 BURGER)
Total Calories: 335; Total Fat: 12g;
Saturated Fat: 3g; Cholesterol: 62mg;
Sodium: 444mg; Potassium: 391mg;
Total Carbohydrate: 29g; Fiber: 2g;
Sugars: 5g; Protein: 30g

1. In a large bowl, mix together the ground turkey breast, two-thirds of the minced garlic, the red onion, spinach, parsley, cumin, oregano, salt, and pepper. Form the mixture into 4 patties.

2. In a nonstick skillet over medium-high heat, heat the olive oil until it shimmers.

3. Add the patties. Cook until browned on both sides, about 7 minutes total. Turn off the heat.

4. Sprinkle the feta on the turkey burgers. Cover the skillet, remove from the heat, and let sit while you prepare the rest of the meal.

5. In a small bowl, stir together the cucumber, dill, lemon juice, yogurt, and remaining garlic. Spread the cucumber mixture on the buns. Add the turkey burgers. Top with the tomato slices, arugula, and remaining bun half.

PREPARATION TIP: After you grate the onion, wrap it in a clean tea towel and wring the water out over the sink to remove as much moisture as possible. This results in a better burger texture.

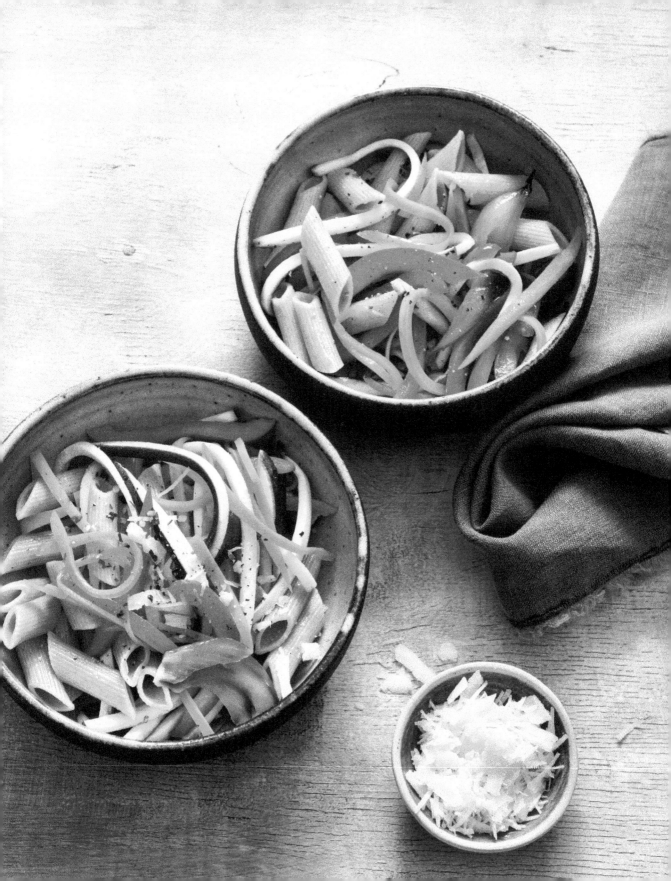

CHAPTER 6

Curried Lentils

SERVES 4   PREP TIME: 10 MINUTES   COOK TIME: 30 MINUTES

DIABETES FRIENDLY • GLUTEN FREE • VEGAN

Lentils are warm and satisfying, and an excellent source of vegetarian protein and fiber. Serve this spicy stew on top of ½ cup cooked brown rice or quinoa. This freezes well, so a double batch can keep you eating for several days; freeze in single servings (1½ cups) for up to 6 months and reheat in the microwave.

2 tablespoons extra-virgin olive oil

1 onion, chopped

2 carrots, chopped

1 red bell pepper, seeded and chopped

3 garlic cloves, minced

2 tablespoons curry powder

1 teaspoon ground turmeric

¼ teaspoon sea salt

4 cups low-sodium vegetable broth

1½ cups dried lentils

PER SERVING (1½ CUPS)
Total Calories: 346; Total Fat: 9g;
Saturated Fat: 1g; Cholesterol: 0mg;
Sodium: 317mg; Potassium: 865mg;
Total Carbohydrate: 51g; Fiber: 24g;
Sugars: 8g; Protein: 19g

1. In a large pot over medium-high heat, heat the olive oil until it shimmers.

2. Add the onion, carrots, and red bell pepper. Cook for about 5 minutes, stirring occasionally, until the vegetables begin to soften.

3. Add the garlic, curry powder, turmeric, and salt. Cook for 1 minute, stirring.

4. Stir in the vegetable broth and lentils. Bring to a boil. Reduce the heat to medium. Simmer, uncovered, for about 20 minutes, stirring occasionally, or until the lentils reach your desired texture.

PREPARATION TIP: If you prefer a creamier curry, stir in up to ¼ cup lite coconut milk just before serving.

Black Bean and Veggie Burritos

SERVES 4   PREP TIME: 10 MINUTES   COOK TIME: 15 MINUTES

DIABETES FRIENDLY • VEGETARIAN • **KIDNEY FRIENDLY**

Adding crunchy slaw to these burritos adds textural contrast, flavor, and vitamin C. These burritos are delicious warm or cold, and you can refrigerate them, tightly wrapped, for up to 5 days for meals in a hurry.

4 (8-inch) whole-wheat tortillas

2 tablespoons extra-virgin olive oil

1 onion, chopped

1 jalapeño pepper, seeded and chopped

1 (15.5-ounce) can low-sodium black beans, drained

1 teaspoon chili powder

½ teaspoon ground cumin

½ cup shredded pepper Jack cheese

1 red bell pepper, seeded and thinly sliced

1 cup shredded cabbage

¼ cup chopped fresh cilantro

4 scallions, white and green parts, thinly sliced

1 recipe Greek Yogurt Southwestern Dressing (page 152)

PER SERVING (1 BURRITO)
Total Calories: 395; Total Fat: 15g;
Saturated Fat: 4g; Cholesterol: 15mg;
Sodium: 376mg; Potassium: 304mg;
Total Carbohydrate: 51g; Fiber: 9g;
Sugars: 9g; Protein: 18g

1. Preheat the oven to 350°F.

2. Wrap the tortillas in aluminum foil and place in the oven for 7 to 10 minutes until warmed through.

3. Meanwhile, in a saucepan over medium-high heat, heat the olive oil until it shimmers.

4. Add the onion and jalapeño. Cook for 5 to 7 minutes, stirring occasionally, until the vegetables are soft.

5. Add the black beans, chili powder, and cumin. Cook for about 2 minutes, stirring, until the beans are warm. Remove from the heat.

6. Using a potato masher, mash the beans. Stir in the cheese. Cover the pan and set aside.

7. In a medium bowl, combine the red bell pepper, cabbage, cilantro, scallions, and dressing. Toss to mix.

8. Spread one-fourth of the bean mixture (about ½ cup) on each warmed tortilla. Top with the slaw and wrap into a burrito.

PREPARATION TIP: To time this recipe well, have all your ingredients measured and prepped before you start cooking.

Bell Pepper and Tofu Stir-Fry

SERVES 4   PREP TIME: 10 MINUTES   COOK TIME: 15 MINUTES

DIABETES FRIENDLY • KIDNEY FRIENDLY • VEGAN

Stir-fries are versatile, quick, and easy. Add your favorite vegetables to satisfy your individual taste. To save time, grab some pre-chopped vegetables from the produce section at your local grocery store or opt for a bag of mixed frozen peppers. The stir-fry freezes well—for up to 6 months—or will keep refrigerated, for up to 5 days. Serve with brown rice.

2 tablespoons extra-virgin olive oil

6 scallions, white and green parts, chopped

1 red bell pepper, seeded and sliced

1 green bell pepper, seeded and sliced

1 orange bell pepper, seeded and sliced

12 ounces extra-firm tofu, patted dry and cut into ½-inch pieces

1 recipe Ginger Stir-Fry Sauce (page 153)

PER SERVING (ABOUT 2 CUPS)
Total Calories: 192; Total Fat: 11g;
Saturated Fat: 1g; Cholesterol: 0mg;
Sodium: 161mg; Potassium: 62mg;
Total Carbohydrate: 16g; Fiber: 3g;
Sugars: 7g; Protein: 10g

1. In a large skillet or wok over medium-high heat, heat the olive oil until it shimmers.
2. Add the scallions, red, green, and orange bell peppers, and tofu. Cook for 5 to 7 minutes, stirring, until the vegetables begin to soften.
3. Stir in the stir-fry sauce. Continue cooking and stirring until the sauce thickens slightly, about 2 minutes.

VARIATION TIP: Omit the green and orange bell pepper and add 2 cups chopped broccoli or broccolini instead.

White Bean Chili

SERVES 4   PREP TIME: 10 MINUTES   COOK TIME: 20 MINUTES

DIABETES FRIENDLY • GLUTEN FREE • KIDNEY FRIENDLY • VEGAN

Serve this hearty chili with brown rice or whole-wheat tortillas. White beans are excellent at soaking up the flavors of the foods they are cooked with and they freeze well. Make a double batch and freeze for up to 6 months, or refrigerate for up to 5 days. Reheat on the stove top or in the microwave.

2 tablespoons extra-virgin olive oil

1 red onion, finely chopped

1 red bell pepper, finely chopped

3 garlic cloves, minced

1 (15.5-ounce) can low-sodium white beans, drained and rinsed

2 cups low-sodium vegetable broth, or water

2 tablespoons chili powder

½ teaspoon sea salt

½ teaspoon dried oregano

1 teaspoon ground cumin

Pinch cayenne pepper (optional)

1 avocado, peeled, pitted, and chopped

1. In a large pot over medium-high heat, heat the olive oil until it shimmers.

2. Add the red onion and red bell pepper. Cook for 5 to 7 minutes, stirring, until the vegetables begin to soften.

3. Add the garlic. Cook for 30 seconds, stirring constantly.

4. Add the white beans, vegetable broth, chili powder, salt, oregano, cumin, and cayenne (if using). Bring to a boil. Reduce the heat to medium and simmer, stirring occasionally, for 5 minutes. Serve topped with the chopped avocado.

PER SERVING (ABOUT 2 CUPS)
Total Calories: 243; Total Fat: 14g; Saturated Fat: 2g; Cholesterol: 0mg; Sodium: 365mg; Potassium: 324mg; Total Carbohydrate: 25g; Fiber: 8g; Sugars: 3g; Protein: 7g

PREPARATION TIP: Garnish with up to 1 tablespoon per serving of low-fat sour cream or plain yogurt and commercially prepared low-sodium salsa.

Sweet Potato Hash with Swiss Chard and Poached Eggs

SERVES 2 PREP TIME: 10 MINUTES COOK TIME: 20 MINUTES

DIABETES FRIENDLY • KIDNEY FRIENDLY • VEGETARIAN

This makes a warm and nutritious meatless meal. It's also a delicious vegetarian breakfast and a great way to add more veggies to your meals. It doesn't keep well in the fridge or freezer, so it's best to make this on demand.

2 tablespoons extra-virgin olive oil

1 yellow onion, chopped

1½ cups cubed (½-inch pieces) unpeeled sweet potato

2 cups chopped stemmed Swiss chard

½ teaspoon ground turmeric

⅛ teaspoon sea salt

⅛ teaspoon ground black pepper

2 large eggs

PER SERVING (ABOUT 1 CUP HASH, 1 EGG)
Total Calories: 333; Total Fat: 19g;
Saturated Fat: 4g; Cholesterol: 211mg;
Sodium: 585mg; Potassium: 510mg;
Total Carbohydrate: 32g; Fiber: 8g;
Sugars: 9g; Protein: 11g

1. In a large nonstick skillet over medium-high heat, heat the olive oil until it shimmers.

2. Add the onion and sweet potato. Cook for about 10 minutes, stirring occasionally, until the vegetables soften.

3. Add the Swiss chard, turmeric, salt, and pepper. Continue to cook for 5 minutes more, stirring occasionally.

4. While the vegetables cook, poach the eggs. Add the eggs to simmering water (see cooking tip) and cook for 2 minutes on the heat. Remove from the heat and let sit, uncovered, for about 8 minutes until the yolks begin to set. Serve the eggs over the hash.

COOKING TIP: To make perfectly poached eggs, crack each egg into its own ramekin. In a saucepan over medium heat, bring 3 to 4 cups water and 1 teaspoon white vinegar to a simmer. Using a wooden spoon, swirl the water. As the water swirls, hold the ramekin just above the water's surface and slip the egg into the swirling water. Add the remaining egg in the same way. Carefully spoon water from the pan over the eggs.

Pasta Primavera

SERVES 4   PREP TIME: 10 MINUTES   COOK TIME: 20 MINUTES

DIABETES FRIENDLY • KIDNEY FRIENDLY • VEGAN OPTION • VEGETARIAN

Primavera is a fresh vegetable–based sauce that's perfect on pasta. Cut the vegetables into thin strips using a vegetable peeler to obtain the right texture and speed up the cooking. If you store this, keep the pasta separate from the sauce and mix just before serving.

2 tablespoons extra-virgin olive oil

1 red onion, thinly sliced

1 red bell pepper, thinly sliced

2 carrots, cut into strips

1 zucchini cut into strips

3 garlic cloves, minced

¼ teaspoon sea salt

¼ teaspoon freshly ground black pepper

Pinch red pepper flakes

4 ounces whole-wheat penne pasta, cooked according to the package directions and drained

1½ cups cherry tomatoes, halved

¼ cup grated Parmesan cheese (omit for vegan option)

PER SERVING (ABOUT 2 CUPS)
Total Calories: 223; Total Fat: 10g;
Saturated Fat: 2g; Cholesterol: 5mg;
Sodium: 259mg; Potassium: 440mg;
Total Carbohydrate: 33g; Fiber: 6g;
Sugars: 3g; Protein: 7g

1. In a large pot over medium-high heat, heat the olive oil until it shimmers.

2. Add the red onion, red bell pepper, carrots, and zucchini. Cook for 5 to 7 minutes, stirring, until the vegetables begin to soften.

3. Add the garlic, salt, pepper, and red pepper flakes. Cook for 30 seconds, stirring constantly.

4. Stir in the cooked pasta and cherry tomatoes. Mix well. Sprinkle with the cheese and serve.

SERVING TIP: Primavera sauce also makes a great topping for fish or chicken. Use ¼ cup to top a 3-ounce serving of grilled skinless chicken or fish.

Sweet-and-Sour Tofu and Veggie Stir-Fry

SERVES 4   PREP TIME: 10 MINUTES   COOK TIME: 15 MINUTES

DIABETES FRIENDLY • KIDNEY FRIENDLY • VEGAN • VEGETARIAN

Serve this with brown rice or quinoa (½ cup cooked per serving) for a simple and satisfying meal. This is a great way to add veggies to your diet, so feel free to add more or change the vegetables here in equal amounts of whatever is seasonally available.

2 tablespoons extra-virgin olive oil

1 yellow onion, thinly sliced

1 green bell pepper, seeded and thinly sliced

1 cup broccoli florets

8 ounces extra firm tofu, cut into ½- to 1-inch pieces

2 garlic cloves, minced

1 cup canned pineapple chunks, drained, with one-fourth of the juice reserved

1 tablespoon rice vinegar

1 tablespoon packed light brown sugar

1 tablespoon low-sodium soy sauce

1 teaspoon grated peeled fresh ginger

½ teaspoon cornstarch

PER SERVING (ABOUT 2 CUPS)
Total Calories: 192; Total Fat: 10g;
Saturated Fat: 1g; Cholesterol: 0mg;
Sodium: 162mg; Potassium: 262mg;
Total Carbohydrate: 21g; Fiber: 3g;
Sugars: 12g; Protein: 8g

1. In a large nonstick skillet over medium-high heat, heat the olive oil until it shimmers.

2. Add the onion, green bell pepper, broccoli, and tofu. Cook for about 7 minutes, stirring occasionally, until the vegetables soften.

3. Add the garlic. Cook for 30 seconds, stirring constantly.

4. Add the pineapple (not the juice). Cook for 2 minutes more, stirring occasionally.

5. In a small bowl, whisk the pineapple juice, vinegar, brown sugar, soy sauce, ginger, and cornstarch until smooth. Add this sauce to the skillet. Bring the mixture to a simmer and cook for about 2 minutes until the sauce thickens, stirring constantly.

VARIATION TIP: Substitute 3 cups edamame for the tofu if you like.

Lentil Barley Stew

SERVES 4   PREP TIME: 10 MINUTES   COOK TIME: 40 MINUTES

GLUTEN FREE OPTION • VEGAN • VEGETARIAN

This stew is a meal by itself. Barley contains gluten, so if you're sensitive to gluten, see the tip for an alternative. If you make a double batch, this freezes well for up to 6 months, or it keeps, refrigerated, for about 5 days.

2 tablespoons extra-virgin olive oil

1 yellow onion, chopped

2 carrots, chopped

2 celery stalks, chopped

1 garlic clove, minced

6 cups low-sodium vegetable broth

1 (15.5-ounce) can no-salt-added crushed tomatoes, drained

1 cup pearl barley

1 cup dried lentils

1 bay leaf

1 tablespoon dried thyme

1 teaspoon ground turmeric

¼ teaspoon freshly ground black pepper

1 tablespoon cornstarch

1 tablespoon water

PER SERVING (ABOUT 2 CUPS)
Total Calories: 468; Total Fat: 9g;
Saturated Fat: 1g; Cholesterol: 0mg;
Sodium: 281mg; Potassium: 1048mg;
Total Carbohydrate: 82g; Fiber: 25g;
Sugars: 11g; Protein: 19g

1. In a large pot over medium-high heat, heat the olive oil until it shimmers.

2. Add the onion, carrots, and celery. Cook for about 5 minutes, stirring occasionally, until the vegetables begin to soften.

3. Add the garlic. Cook for 30 seconds, stirring constantly.

4. Stir in the vegetable broth, tomatoes, barley, lentils, bay leaf, thyme, turmeric, and pepper. Bring to a boil. Reduce the heat to medium-low. Simmer for about 25 minutes, stirring frequently, until the barley and lentils are soft. Remove and discard the bay leaf.

5. In a small bowl, whisk the cornstarch and water until smooth. Stir this slurry into the stew. Cook for about 3 minutes, stirring, until the stew starts to thicken.

PREPARATION TIP: To make this gluten free, replace the barley with 1 cup brown rice. Add the rice to the pot in step 4, but do not add the lentils until the rice has cooked for 15 minutes. Then add the lentils and cook for 25 minutes more until the rice and lentils are tender. Alternatively, omit the barley and stir in cooked brown rice just before serving.

Red Beans and Brown Rice

SERVES 4   PREP TIME: 10 MINUTES   COOK TIME: 15 MINUTES

DIABETES FRIENDLY • GLUTEN FREE • KIDNEY FRIENDLY • VEGAN • VEGETARIAN

Red beans and rice is a flavorful traditional Cajun dish that usually features andouille sausage. This vegan version has the same great Cajun flavors but without the meat. While it is typically slow simmered, using cooked brown rice and canned kidney beans speeds up the process by several hours with the same great flavor you get from the original method of preparation.

2 tablespoons extra-virgin olive oil

1 yellow onion, chopped

1 green bell pepper, seeded and chopped

1 celery stalk, chopped

½ cup low-sodium vegetable broth

1 (15.5-ounce) can low-sodium kidney beans, rinsed and drained

2 cups cooked brown rice

1 teaspoon garlic powder

1 teaspoon dried thyme

½ teaspoon dried oregano

Pinch red pepper flakes

½ teaspoon freshly ground black pepper

2 teaspoons Louisiana hot sauce

1. In a large pot over medium-high heat, heat the olive oil until it shimmers.

2. Add the onion, green bell pepper, and celery. Cook for about 5 minutes, stirring occasionally, until the vegetables begin to soften.

3. Add the vegetable broth, kidney beans, brown rice, garlic powder, thyme, oregano, red pepper flakes, black pepper, and hot sauce. Bring to a simmer. Cook for 5 minutes, stirring occasionally, or until warmed through.

PREPARATION TIP: If you like it spicy, add up to ¼ teaspoon cayenne pepper. It's best to start with a pinch, taste, and add a little more to reach your desired level of heat.

PER SERVING (ABOUT 1 CUP)
Total Calories: 276; Total Fat: 8g;
Saturated Fat: 1g; Cholesterol: 0mg;
Sodium: 98mg; Potassium: 176mg;
Total Carbohydrate: 43g; Fiber: 7g;
Sugars: 3g; Protein: 8g

Lemon Garlic Chickpeas

SERVES 4   PREP TIME: 10 MINUTES   COOK TIME: 15 MINUTES

DIABETES FRIENDLY • GLUTEN FREE • KIDNEY FRIENDLY • VEGAN • VEGETARIAN

Serve this chickpea stew with whole-grain tortillas or have it over ½ cup brown rice. With aromatic Mediterranean flavors, this is a really delicious and quick stew that stores and travels well.

2 tablespoons extra-virgin olive oil

1 red onion, chopped

2 carrots, chopped

6 garlic cloves, minced (see preparation tip)

1 (15.5-ounce) can low-sodium chickpeas, rinsed and drained

1 cup low-sodium vegetable broth

1 teaspoon ground turmeric

Juice of 1 lemon

Zest of 1 lemon

½ teaspoon sea salt

¼ cup chopped fresh Italian parsley

1. In a large pot over medium-high heat, heat the olive oil until it shimmers.
2. Add the red onion and carrots. Cook for about 5 minutes, stirring occasionally, until the vegetables begin to soften.
3. Add the garlic. Cook for 30 seconds, stirring constantly.
4. Add the chickpeas, vegetable broth, turmeric, lemon juice and zest, and salt. Bring to a boil. Reduce the heat to low. Cook for 5 minutes, stirring.
5. Remove from the heat and stir in the parsley.

PER SERVING (ABOUT 1 CUP)
Total Calories: 182; Total Fat: 7g;
Saturated Fat: 1g; Cholesterol: 0mg;
Sodium: 351mg; Potassium: 208mg;
Total Carbohydrate: 24g; Fiber: 6g;
Sugars: 4g; Protein: 6g

VARIATION TIP: You can also replace the chickpeas with an equal amount of white beans if you prefer. If you do, replace the lemon with an equal amount of orange.

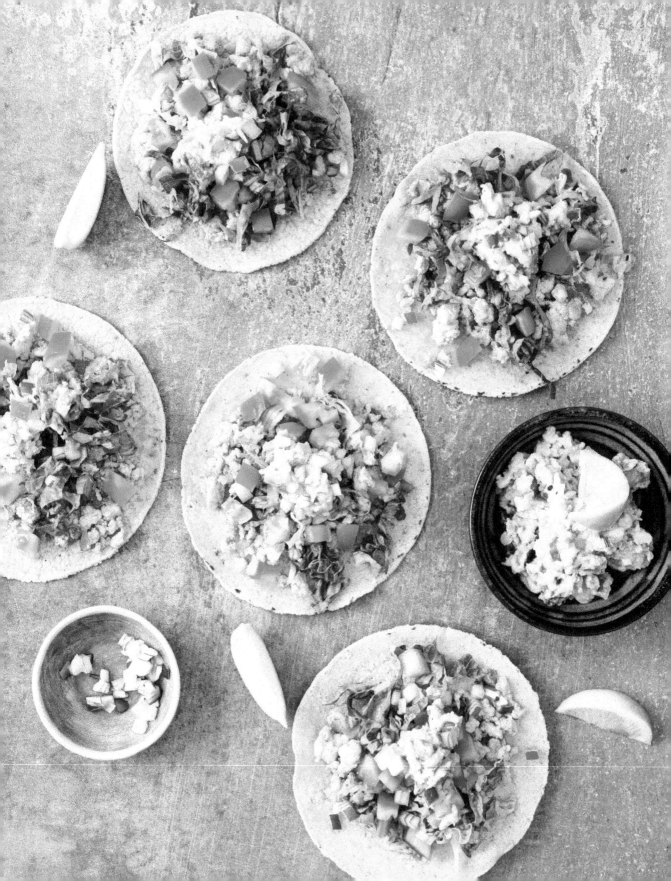

CHAPTER 7

Balsamic Chicken Breast with Brussels Sprouts

SERVES 4   PREP TIME: 10 MINUTES   COOK TIME: 30 MINUTES

DIABETES FRIENDLY • GLUTEN FREE • KIDNEY FRIENDLY

While you can use any aged balsamic vinegar here, a high-quality product delivers the best flavor. Anything barrel aged is usually flavorful and a good quality. To make the Brussels sprouts, trim the ends completely and separate the leaves from the heads, which will happen naturally once the ends are trimmed. This trick substantially decreases the time it takes to cook the Brussels sprouts, from 45 minutes to 3 minutes. If that sounds like too much trouble, see the tip.

3 tablespoons extra-virgin olive oil, divided

4 (3-ounce) pieces boneless, skinless chicken breast, pounded to ½-inch thickness between two pieces of parchment paper

½ teaspoon sea salt, divided

¼ teaspoon freshly ground black pepper

½ cup aged balsamic vinegar

2 cups Brussels sprouts, ends removed and leaves separated (see headnote)

Pinch red pepper flakes

PER SERVING (3 OUNCES CHICKEN, ¼ CUP BRUSSELS SPROUTS)
Total Calories: 211; Total Fat: 12g; Saturated Fat: 1g; Cholesterol: 41mg; Sodium: 469mg; Potassium: 171mg; Total Carbohydrate: 8g; Fiber: 2g; Sugars: 5g; Protein: 19g

1. In a large nonstick skillet over medium-high heat, heat 1½ teaspoons of olive oil until it shimmers.

2. Season the chicken with ¼ teaspoon of salt and the pepper. One at a time, cook the chicken pieces for about 3 minutes per side until cooked through, adding 1½ teaspoons of olive oil for each piece. Set the chicken aside tented with aluminum foil to keep warm.

3. Add the remaining 1 tablespoon of olive oil to the pan and heat until it shimmers.

4. Add the Brussels sprouts and remaining ¼ teaspoon of salt. Cook for about 3 minutes, stirring occasionally, until the sprouts soften. If you like your Brussels sprouts browned, cook them for an additional 15 minutes, stirring occasionally, or until they reach your desired level of doneness.

5. Add the balsamic vinegar. Bring to a simmer. Add the chicken, and turn it in the sprouts and vinegar several times to coat. Serve the chicken with the sprouts spooned over the top.

PREPARATION TIP: You can also roast Brussels sprouts separately from the chicken. Preheat the oven to 400°F. Trim the ends off the sprouts and halve them lengthwise. Place in a single layer, cut-side down, on a rimmed baking sheet and drizzle with 1 tablespoon of olive oil. Roast for 45 to 50 minutes, or until browned. After cooking the chicken in the skillet, add the balsamic vinegar and red pepper flakes and bring to a simmer. Simmer for about 5 minutes until reduced by half. Turn each piece of chicken in the warm balsamic vinegar to coat it. Serve the warmed balsamic vinegar spooned over the chicken and Brussels sprouts.

Turkey with Wild Rice and Kale

SERVES 4 PREP TIME: 10 MINUTES   COOK TIME: 20 MINUTES

DIABETES FRIENDLY • GLUTEN FREE • KIDNEY FRIENDLY

Cook your wild rice ahead according to the package instructions to make this meal come together quickly. Many people are surprised to learn wild rice isn't actually rice; it's a grass. It's an excellent source of vitamin B_6 and magnesium, and it adds nice flavor and texture to dishes.

2 tablespoons extra-virgin olive oil

12 ounces 93% lean ground turkey breast

2 cups chopped stemmed kale

1 red onion, chopped

Juice of 1 lemon

1 teaspoon ground turmeric

½ teaspoon sea salt

2 cups cooked wild rice

2 garlic cloves, minced

PER SERVING (ABOUT 2 CUPS)
Total Calories: 358; Total Fat: 15g;
Saturated Fat: 3g; Cholesterol: 60mg;
Sodium: 364mg; Potassium: 78mg;
Total Carbohydrate: 41g; Fiber: 4g;
Sugars: 1g; Protein: 22g

1. In a large nonstick skillet over medium-high heat, heat the olive oil until it shimmers.
2. Add the ground turkey breast. Cook for about 5 minutes, stirring and crumbling with a spoon, until it starts to brown.
3. Add the kale. Cook for about 5 minutes more, stirring, until the kale softens.
4. Add the red onion, lemon juice, turmeric, salt, and wild rice. Cook for 5 minutes, stirring occasionally.
5. Add the garlic. Cook for 30 seconds, stirring.

PREPARATION TIP: Wild rice takes about 45 minutes to cook, so cooking a batch and freezing it in 1-cup servings can save you time for weekday meals. Thaw in the refrigerator or microwave before adding to this dish.

Asian Ground Turkey and Bok Choy Stir-Fry

SERVES 4   PREP TIME: 10 MINUTES   COOK TIME: 15 MINUTES

DIABETES FRIENDLY • KIDNEY FRIENDLY

If you can get baby bok choy for this dish, all you need to do is halve it lengthwise to prep it. Otherwise, chop the bok choy into bite-size pieces before adding it to the stir-fry. Bok choy adds vitamin C and a nutty, slightly bitter flavor that's delicious in this simple stir-fry. Serve with ½ cup brown rice, if you choose.

2 tablespoons extra-virgin olive oil

12 ounces 99% extra-lean ground turkey breast

6 scallions, white and green parts, sliced, plus more for garnishing (optional)

3 cups chopped bok choy

1 recipe Ginger Stir-Fry Sauce (page 153)

2 tablespoons sesame seeds, toasted

PER SERVING (ABOUT 1 CUP)
Total Calories: 211; Total Fat: 11g;
Saturated Fat: 2g; Cholesterol: 41mg;
Sodium: 236mg; Potassium: 257mg;
Total Carbohydrate: 6g; Fiber: 1g;
Sugars: 1g; Protein: 23g

1. In a large nonstick skillet over medium-high heat, heat the olive oil until it shimmers.

2. Add the ground turkey breast. Cook for about 5 minutes, stirring and crumbling with a spoon, until it starts to brown.

3. Add the scallions and bok choy. Cook for about 3 minutes, stirring, until the vegetables begin to soften.

4. Add the stir-fry sauce. Cook for about 2 minutes more, stirring, until it begins to thicken.

5. Garnish with the sesame seeds and additional scallions, if desired.

INGREDIENT TIP: Be sure to rinse bok choy well as it tends to be sandy. Can't find bok choy? Replace it with 3 cups shredded green cabbage or coleslaw mix.

Spaghetti with Chicken Meatballs and Marinara

SERVES 4   PREP TIME: 15 MINUTES   COOK TIME: 35 MINUTES

DIABETES FRIENDLY • GLUTEN FREE OPTION • KIDNEY FRIENDLY

If you're in need of a classic comfort meal, you can't go wrong with spaghetti and meatballs. These chicken meatballs are flavorful and the sauce is lightly spicy. Store the sauce, meatballs, and spaghetti separately if you plan to make it and take it, and combine after reheating.

½ cup whole-grain bread crumbs

½ cup low-fat milk

12 ounces ground chicken breast

½ onion, finely chopped

1 large egg, beaten

1 teaspoon dried Italian seasoning

1 teaspoon garlic powder

½ teaspoon sea salt

⅛ teaspoon freshly ground black pepper

Pinch red pepper flakes

2 tablespoons extra-virgin olive oil

1 recipe Basic Marinara Sauce (page 155)

4 ounces whole-wheat spaghetti, cooked according to the package instructions and drained

1. In a large bowl, stir together the bread crumbs and milk. Let sit for 10 minutes.

2. To the bread crumb mixture, add the ground chicken breast, onion, egg, Italian seasoning, garlic powder, salt, black pepper, and red pepper flakes. Mix to combine. Form the mixture into 16 meatballs.

3. In a large nonstick skillet over medium-high heat, heat the olive oil until it shimmers.

4. Working in batches, cook the meatballs for about 15 minutes, turning occasionally, until they are cooked through.

PER SERVING (ABOUT 1 OUNCE PASTA, ½ CUP MARINARA, 4 MEATBALLS)
Total Calories: 433; Total Fat: 17g; Saturated Fat: 3g; Cholesterol: 109mg; Sodium: 410mg; Potassium: 513mg; Total Carbohydrate: 39g; Fiber: 6g; Sugars: 7g; Protein: 28g

5. Add the marinara sauce to the meatballs and bring to a simmer. Simmer for about 5 minutes, stirring occasionally and turning the meatballs to coat.

6. Spoon the meatballs and sauce over the spaghetti.

PREPARATION TIP: To make this gluten free, choose gluten-free spaghetti or make zucchini noodles using a spiralizer or by peeling the zucchini in strips with a vegetable peeler and using a sharp knife to cut the strips into noodles. Also use gluten-free bread crumbs in the meatballs.

Turkey Piccata with Whole-Wheat Penne

SERVES 4   PREP TIME: 10 MINUTES   COOK TIME: 30 MINUTES

DIABETES FRIENDLY • GLUTEN FREE OPTION • KIDNEY FRIENDLY

Capers are salty and a little acidic, and add a nice counterpoint to the turkey and pasta. To prepare the capers before adding them to the sauce, remove them from the brine, put them in a colander or fine-mesh sieve, and rinse them thoroughly to remove as much of the salt from the surface as possible.

3 tablespoons whole-wheat flour

¼ teaspoon sea salt

¼ teaspoon freshly ground black pepper

4 (3-ounce) turkey breast cutlets, pounded to ¼- to ½-inch thickness between two pieces of parchment paper

3 tablespoons extra-virgin olive oil, divided

2 tablespoons minced shallot

2 garlic cloves, sliced

1 cup low-sodium chicken broth, or Poultry Broth (page 148)

Juice of 1 lemon

1 tablespoon capers, drained and rinsed

2 tablespoons chopped fresh Italian parsley

4 ounces whole-wheat penne pasta, cooked according to the package directions and drained

PER SERVING (ABOUT 3 OUNCES TURKEY, 1 OUNCE PASTA)
Total Calories: 322; Total Fat: 12g; Saturated Fat: 1g; Cholesterol: 52mg; Sodium: 310mg; Potassium: 138mg; Total Carbohydrate: 28g; Fiber: 4g; Sugars: 1g; Protein: 26g

1. In a zip-top bag, combine the flour, salt, and pepper. Seal the bag and shake to mix.

2. Add the turkey cutlets. Seal the bag and shake to coat.

3. In a nonstick skillet over medium-high heat, heat 1½ teaspoons of olive oil until it shimmers.

4. One at a time, tap off any excess flour and add the turkey cutlets to the hot oil. Cook for about 5 minutes, turning once halfway through, until opaque. Set each cooked piece aside on a platter tented with aluminum foil to keep warm. Continue with the remaining cutlets, adding an additional 1½ teaspoons of olive oil for each.

5. Add the remaining 1 tablespoon of olive oil to the skillet and heat until it shimmers.

6. Add the shallot and garlic. Cook for about 3 minutes, stirring, until the vegetables soften.

7. Stir in the chicken broth and lemon juice, scraping up any browned bits from the bottom of the skillet. Add the capers. Cook for 1 to 2 minutes, stirring, until the liquid thickens. Stir in the parsley.

8. Return the turkey to the skillet, turning each piece to coat.

9. Serve the turkey and sauce spooned over the pasta.

INGREDIENT TIP: Capers are the buds of the *capparis spinose* plant that have been brined. They can typically be found in small jars near the olives and pickles in the grocery store.

PREPARATION TIP: To make this gluten free, choose a gluten-free pasta and a gluten-free flour, such as brown rice flour.

Slow-Cooker Turkey Breast with Root Vegetables

SERVES 5   PREP TIME: 15 MINUTES   COOK TIME: 8 HOURS

DIABETES FRIENDLY • GLUTEN FREE

Cook the turkey breast with the skin on to retain moisture but remove it before serving. This recipe calls for a 4-pound, bone-in turkey breast. There's about 4 ounces of meat per pound of turkey breast, so calculate the number of meat servings based on the size of the breast you find. You can add more root veggies for larger breasts.

2 large sweet potatoes, scrubbed and cut into 1-inch pieces

2 fennel bulbs, cored and cut into 1-inch pieces (see cooking tip, page 119)

2 red onions, cut into 1-inch pieces

4 carrots, cut into 1-inch pieces

½ cup low-sodium chicken broth, or Poultry Broth (page 148)

½ teaspoon sea salt

¼ teaspoon freshly ground black pepper

1 teaspoon garlic powder

1 teaspoon dried thyme

1 (4-pound) bone-in, skin-on turkey breast

1. In a slow cooker, arrange the sweet potatoes, fennel, red onions, and carrots.

2. Pour in the chicken broth.

3. In a small bowl, stir together the salt, pepper, garlic powder, and thyme. Spread the seasoning under the skin of the turkey breast. Place the turkey breast in the slow cooker on top of the vegetables.

4. Cover the cooker and set to low heat. Cook for 8 hours. Alternatively, set the cooker to high heat and cook for 5 hours.

INGREDIENT TIP: If you can't find a whole turkey breast, use whole skin-on chicken breasts. Each breast serves about three people.

PER SERVING (ABOUT 3 OUNCES TURKEY, 1 CUP VEGETABLES)
Total Calories: 321; Total Fat: 10g;
Saturated Fat: 2g; Cholesterol: 69mg;
Sodium: 401mg; Potassium: 916mg;
Total Carbohydrate: 31g; Fiber: 7g;
Sugars: 10g; Protein: 28g

Pesto Chicken with Roasted Tomatoes

SERVES 4   PREP TIME: 10 MINUTES   COOK TIME: 1 HOUR

DIABETES FRIENDLY • GLUTEN FREE • KIDNEY FRIENDLY

Serve this with whole-wheat pasta, brown rice, or baked sweet potatoes for a tasty and nutritious meal. Use any leftover chicken in salads for lunches or reheat in the microwave for a delicious meal in a hurry. Remove the skin if you're going to use the leftover chicken in a salad.

3 cups cherry tomatoes, halved

4 boneless, skinless chicken thighs

1 recipe Pesto Sauce (page 154)

PER SERVING (1 THIGH, ½ CUP VEGETABLES)
Total Calories: 335; Total Fat: 24g;
Saturated Fat: 5g; Cholesterol: 70mg;
Sodium: 186mg; Potassium: 299mg;
Total Carbohydrate: 7g; Fiber: 2g;
Sugars: <1g; Protein: 25g

1. Preheat the oven to 375°F.
2. In a rimmed baking dish, spread the cherry tomatoes in an even layer on the bottom.
3. Top with the chicken thighs. Spoon some of the pesto over the top of each thigh.
4. Bake for about 1 hour, until the thigh juices run clear.

PREPARATION TIP: When using skinless thighs, it's a good idea to toss the tomatoes with 2 tablespoons extra-virgin olive oil before adding them to the pan.

Chicken Tacos

SERVES 4   PREP TIME: 15 MINUTES   COOK TIME: 15 MINUTES

DIABETES FRIENDLY • GLUTEN FREE • KIDNEY FRIENDLY

Tacos are always a popular meal because they're quick, easy, and tasty. This version uses ground chicken breast (although you can substitute ground turkey breast) and homemade taco seasoning so you can control the sodium levels in your seasoning blend. There's also a quick guacamole to bring a real party feel to your taco meal.

For the tacos

8 soft corn tortillas

2 tablespoons extra-virgin olive oil

12 ounces ground chicken breast

½ cup water

1 teaspoon garlic powder

1 tablespoon chili powder

1 teaspoon ground coriander

½ teaspoon ground cumin

¼ teaspoon sea salt

Pinch cayenne pepper

1 cup shredded lettuce

1 tomato, chopped

For the guacamole

1 avocado, peeled, pitted, and cubed

1 tablespoon freshly squeezed lime juice

1 tablespoon minced red onion

¼ teaspoon sea salt

PER SERVING (2 TACOS, 2 TBSP GUACAMOLE)
Total Calories: 335; Total Fat: 16g;
Saturated Fat: 2g; Cholesterol: 55mg;
Sodium: 368mg; Potassium: 330mg;
Total Carbohydrate: 28g; Fiber: 6g;
Sugars: 2g; Protein: 22g

To make the tacos

1. Preheat the oven to 350°F.
2. Wrap the corn tortillas in aluminum foil and place them in the oven for about 7 minutes until warmed.
3. Meanwhile, in a nonstick skillet over medium-high heat, heat the olive oil until it shimmers.
4. Add the ground chicken breast. Cook for about 7 minutes, stirring and crumbling with a spoon, until browned.
5. Add the water, garlic powder, chili powder, coriander, cumin, salt, and cayenne. Bring to a simmer. Reduce the heat to low and simmer for 5 minutes.

To make the guacamole

1. In a small bowl, using a fork, mash the avocado with the lime juice, red onion, and salt.
2. To assemble, spoon the meat onto the warmed tortillas and top with the guacamole, lettuce, and tomato.

VARIATION TIP: Try the Greek Yogurt Southwestern Dressing (page 152) on theses tacos.

Chicken Satay with Peanut Sauce

SERVES 4   PREP TIME: 15 MINUTES, PLUS MARINATING TIME   COOK TIME: 10 MINUTES

DIABETES FRIENDLY • GLUTEN FREE OPTION • KIDNEY FRIENDLY

It's really easy to make homemade peanut sauce, which is delicious on this chicken satay or with other meats as well. Serve with a salad and brown rice to complete the meal. While most chicken satay comes grilled on skewers, it's just as easy here to bake it without the skewers—and it makes it easier to eat, too.

For the satay

2 tablespoons low-sodium soy sauce, or gluten-free tamari

Juice of 2 limes

3 garlic cloves, minced

1 tablespoon grated peeled fresh ginger

½ teaspoon ground coriander

12 ounces boneless, skinless chicken breast, cut into ½-inch strips

For the peanut sauce

6 scallions, white and green parts, finely chopped

½ cup no-salt-added all-natural peanut butter

¼ cup lite coconut milk

2 tablespoons fresh cilantro leaves

1 garlic clove, minced

1 tablespoon low-sodium soy sauce

2 teaspoons freshly squeezed lime juice

1 teaspoon grated peeled fresh ginger

1 teaspoon sesame oil

Pinch red pepper flakes

PER SERVING (3 OUNCES)
Total Calories: 415; Total Fat: 30g;
Saturated Fat: 5g; Cholesterol: 41mg;
Sodium: 605mg; Potassium: 327mg;
Total Carbohydrate: 14g; Fiber: 4g;
Sugars: 2g; Protein: 27g

To make the satay

1. In a blender or food processor, combine the soy sauce, lime juice, garlic, ginger, and coriander. Blend until smooth. Pour into a zip-top bag. Add the chicken, seal the bag, and refrigerate to marinate for 4 hours.

2. Preheat the broiler to its highest setting and set an oven rack in its highest position.

3. Remove the chicken from the marinade and place it on a broiler pan. Broil for 5 to 7 minutes until the chicken juices run clear.

To make the peanut sauce

In a blender or food processor, combine the scallions, peanut butter, coconut milk, cilantro, garlic, soy sauce, lime juice, ginger, sesame oil, and red pepper flakes. Blend until smooth. Serve the peanut sauce spooned over the chicken satay.

PREPARATION TIP: If you want to grill the satay, soak wooden skewers in water while you marinate the chicken. Thread the chicken onto the skewers. Preheat the grill to high and brush it with oil. Grill the skewers for about 3 minutes per side and serve with the peanut sauce.

Southwestern Buddha Bowl

SERVES 4   PREP TIME: 15 MINUTES, PLUS MARINATING TIME   COOK TIME: 10 MINUTES

DIABETES FRIENDLY • GLUTEN FREE • KIDNEY FRIENDLY

Buddha bowls are grain-based bowls with some type of protein and lots of veggies. While they typically have Asian flavors, these are Southwestern— think of it like a burrito but without the tortilla. What's nice about this dish is how quickly the bowls come together and how easy they are to customize with whatever you have available in your fridge.

Juice of 2 limes

6 scallions, white and green parts, roughly chopped

¼ cup fresh cilantro leaves

2 garlic cloves, minced

1 teaspoon chili powder

½ teaspoon sea salt

3 tablespoons extra-virgin olive oil, divided

12 ounces boneless, skinless chicken breast, cut into ½-inch strips

2 cups cooked brown rice

1 avocado, peeled, pitted, and chopped

1 tomato, chopped

¼ cup plain low-fat Greek yogurt

PER SERVING (3 OUNCES CHICKEN, ½ CUP BROWN RICE)
Total Calories: 392; Total Fat: 19g;
Saturated Fat: 3g; Cholesterol: 43mg;
Sodium: 467mg; Potassium: 461mg;
Total Carbohydrate: 33g; Fiber: 7g;
Sugars: 2g; Protein: 23g

1. In a blender or food processor, combine the lime juice, scallions, cilantro, garlic, chili powder, salt, and 2 tablespoons of olive oil. Process until smooth. Reserve 2 tablespoons of the marinade and pour the rest into a zip-top bag. Add the chicken, seal the bag, and toss to coat. Refrigerate to marinate for at least 4 hours.

2. In a large nonstick skillet over medium-high heat, heat the remaining 1 tablespoon of olive oil until it shimmers.

3. Remove the chicken from the marinade, discarding the bag and its contents, and pat it dry. Carefully add it to the hot oil. Cook for 5 to 7 minutes until opaque.

4. Add the reserved marinade. Cook for 1 minute more, stirring.

5. To assemble the bowls, place ½ cup of rice into each bowl. Top with the chicken, avocado, tomato, and a dollop of yogurt.

INGREDIENT TIP: Look for precooked brown rice in the freezer section of your local grocery store to save some prep time.

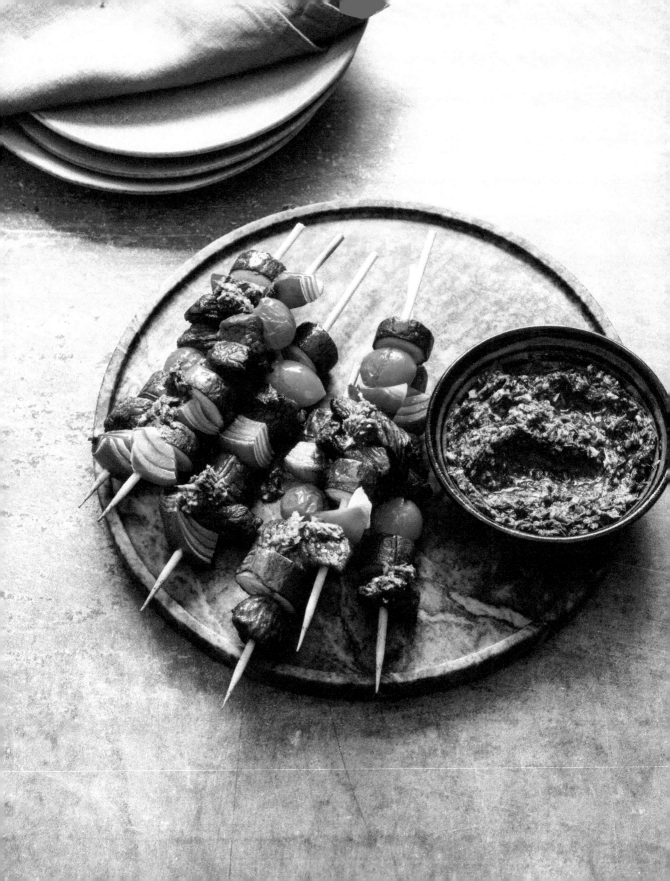

CHAPTER 8

Pork Tenderloin and Greens with Mustard Sauce

SERVES 4   PREP TIME: 10 MINUTES, PLUS MARINATING TIME   COOK TIME: 35 MINUTES

DIABETES FRIENDLY • GLUTEN FREE • KIDNEY FRIENDLY

Pork tenderloin is an excellent lean meat for people watching their fat intake. Some pork tenderloins are sold pre-marinated, which are high in sodium—read the label to make sure all you're buying is tenderloin. You can replace the Swiss chard with kale, mustard greens, collard greens, or spinach, if you wish.

¼ cup apple cider vinegar

2 tablespoons Dijon mustard

1 shallot, minced

1 tablespoon dried thyme

1 (12-ounce) pork tenderloin

2 tablespoons extra-virgin olive oil

4 cups chopped stemmed Swiss chard

1 garlic clove, minced

PER SERVING (3 OUNCES TENDERLOIN, ½ CUP GREENS)
Total Calories: 276; Total Fat: 14g;
Saturated Fat: 3g; Cholesterol: 67mg;
Sodium: 540mg; Potassium: 535mg;
Total Carbohydrate: 8g; Fiber: 4g;
Sugars: 2g; Protein: 28g

1. In a small bowl, whisk the vinegar, mustard, shallot, and thyme. Reserve 1 tablespoon of the marinade and pour the rest in a zip-top bag. Add the tenderloin to the marinade in the bag. Seal the bag and coat the tenderloin with the marinade. Refrigerate to marinate for 4 hours.

2. Preheat the oven to 400°F.

3. Remove the tenderloin from the marinade and put it in a roasting pan. Roast, uncovered, for 25 to 30 minutes, or until the internal temperature reaches 145°F. Let rest, tented with aluminum foil, for 15 minutes.

4. In a large skillet over medium-high heat, heat the olive oil until it shimmers.

5. Add the Swiss chard. Cook for about 4 minutes, stirring occasionally, until soft. Add the garlic. Cook for 30 seconds, stirring constantly.

6. Add the reserved marinade to the Swiss chard. Cook for 1 minute more, stirring.

7. Slice the tenderloin and serve over the chard.

INGREDIENT TIP: If you don't have Dijon mustard, add 2 tablespoons dried mustard to the marinade instead..

Pork Tenderloin Fajitas with Guacamole

SERVES 4   PREP TIME: 10 MINUTES, PLUS MARINATING TIME   COOK TIME: 25 MINUTES

DIABETES FRIENDLY • GLUTEN FREE OPTION

The secret with these fajitas is reserving part of the marinade to mix with the meat and veggies at the end. This adds a tremendous amount of flavor to these delicious fajitas. If you like sour cream with your fajitas, feel free to add a tablespoon of plain low-fat Greek yogurt to each as a healthier alternative.

Juice of 3 limes, divided

3 tablespoons extra-virgin olive oil, divided

6 scallions, white and green parts, minced

6 garlic cloves, minced, divided

¼ cup fresh cilantro leaves

½ jalapeño pepper, seeded and minced

1 (12-ounce) pork tenderloin, halved lengthwise and pounded to an even ¾- to 1-inch thickness

4 (8-inch) whole-wheat tortillas

1 green bell pepper, thinly sliced

1 red bell pepper, thinly sliced

1 yellow onion, thinly sliced

1 avocado, peeled, pitted, and cubed

¼ teaspoon sea salt

1. In a blender or food processor, combine the juice of 2 limes, 2 tablespoons of olive oil, the scallions, 5 garlic cloves, cilantro, and jalapeño. Blend until a paste forms. Reserve 1 tablespoon of the marinade. Put the rest in a zip-top bag and add the pork tenderloin. Seal the bag and turn the pork to coat. Refrigerate to marinate for 2 to 4 hours.

2. Preheat the oven to 350°F.

3. Wrap the tortillas in aluminum foil and place them in the oven for 10 minutes until warm.

4. In a large skillet over medium-high heat, heat the remaining 2 tablespoons of olive oil until it shimmers.

PER SERVING (3 OUNCES MEAT, 1 TORTILLA, ½ CUP VEGETABLES)
Total Calories: 518; Total Fat: 27g;
Saturated Fat: 5g; Cholesterol: 67mg;
Sodium: 433mg; Potassium: 906mg;
Total Carbohydrate: 37g; Fiber: 9g;
Sugars: 6g; Protein: 32g

5. Remove the pork from the marinade and use a paper towel to wipe any excess marinade off the surface. Carefully add the pork to the hot oil. Cook for 3 to 4 minutes per side until it reaches an internal temperature of 145°F. Remove and let rest while you cook the vegetables.

6. Return the skillet to the heat and add the green and red bell peppers and onion. Cook for about 5 minutes, stirring occasionally, until the vegetables soften.

7. Slice the pork into 1-inch-thick slices and return them to the pan. Add the reserved marinade. Cook for 1 minute, stirring.

8. In a small bowl, mash the avocado with the juice of the remaining 1 lime, the remaining 1 garlic clove, and the salt.

9. To serve, spoon the meat and veggies on the warm tortillas and top with the guacamole.

INGREDIENT TIP: To make this gluten free, serve the fajitas over steamed brown rice, ¼ cup per serving.

Thin-Cut Pork Chops with Gingered Applesauce

SERVES 4   PREP TIME: 10 MINUTES   COOK TIME: 20 MINUTES

DIABETES FRIENDLY • GLUTEN FREE • KIDNEY FRIENDLY

Thin-cut pork chops cook so quickly they don't dry out the way thicker pork chops might. If you don't have the time to make your own applesauce, buy some from the store and modify it (see cooking tip).

4 sweet-tart apples, such as Braeburn or Granny Smith, peeled, cored, and chopped

¾ cup water

2 tablespoons packed light brown sugar

1 tablespoon grated peeled fresh ginger, or 1 teaspoon ground ginger

1 teaspoon dried thyme

½ teaspoon sea salt

¼ teaspoon ground black pepper

4 thin-cut pork chops, trimmed of excess fat

2 tablespoons extra-virgin olive oil

PER SERVING (1 PORK CHOP, ¼ CUP APPLESAUCE)
Total Calories: 325; Total Fat: 15g;
Saturated Fat: 4g; Cholesterol: 44mg;
Sodium: 351mg; Potassium: 488mg;
Total Carbohydrate: 35g; Fiber: 4g;
Sugars: 26g; Protein: 16g

1. In a large pot over medium-high heat, combine the apples, water, brown sugar, and ginger. Cover the pot and cook for 15 to 20 minutes until the apples are soft.

2. Meanwhile, in a small bowl, stir together the thyme, salt, and pepper. Sprinkle the seasoning on the pork chops.

3. In a large skillet over medium-high heat, heat the olive oil until it shimmers.

4. Add the pork chops. Cook for about 3 minutes per side until golden brown.

5. Spoon the applesauce over the pork chops to serve.

COOKING TIP: No time for fresh apple-sauce? Stir 1 tablespoon grated peeled fresh ginger into store-bought unsweetened applesauce.

Hearty Meat Loaf Muffins

SERVES 6   PREP TIME: 10 MINUTES   COOK TIME: 30 MINUTES

DIABETES FRIENDLY • GLUTEN FREE OPTION • KIDNEY FRIENDLY

Making meat loaf muffins means the meat loaf cooks much more quickly than a whole loaf, and they're excellent for portion control. Serve with steamed veggies, such as green beans, and brown rice or roasted baby potatoes for a complete meal. These freeze well in zip-top bags for up to 6 months. Thaw in the fridge and reheat in the microwave.

½ cup whole-wheat bread crumbs

½ cup low-fat milk

9 ounces 95% extra-lean ground beef

9 ounces 93% lean ground turkey

2 tablespoons Dijon mustard

2 carrots, grated

1 small zucchini, grated

½ red onion, finely chopped

1 tablespoon dried thyme

1 teaspoon garlic powder

¼ teaspoon sea salt

¼ teaspoon freshly ground black pepper

PER SERVING (2 MUFFINS)
Total Calories: 191; Total Fat: 8g;
Saturated Fat: 3g; Cholesterol: 61mg;
Sodium: 313mg; Potassium: 203mg;
Total Carbohydrate: 10g; Fiber: 2g;
Sugars: 3g; Protein: 18g

1. Preheat the oven to 350°F.
2. In a large bowl, combine the bread crumbs and milk. Let sit for 5 minutes.
3. To the bread crumb mixture, add the ground beef, ground turkey, mustard, carrots, zucchini, red onion, thyme, garlic powder, salt, and pepper. Mix well. Press the meat mixture into a 12-cup muffin tin, filling the wells.
4. Bake for 25 to 30 minutes until the internal temperature reaches 160°F.

INGREDIENT TIP: To make this gluten free, replace the bread crumbs with ½ cup gluten-free oats.

Sirloin Tips with Mushrooms and Brown Rice

SERVES 6   PREP TIME: 10 MINUTES   COOK TIME: 30 MINUTES

DIABETES FRIENDLY • KIDNEY FRIENDLY

Sirloin tips are a flavorful, tender cut of meat. Cut them into cubes so they'll cook quickly without toughening up. The secret to adding even more flavor is cooking the mushrooms and onion until deeply browned and making sure the meat browns well, too. This adds savoriness to the finished dish.

4 tablespoons extra-virgin olive oil, divided

12 ounces sirloin tips, cut into 1-inch cubes

¼ teaspoon sea salt

¼ teaspoon freshly ground black pepper

8 ounces cremini mushrooms, quartered

1 red onion, chopped

3 garlic cloves, minced

2 cups low-sodium chicken broth

2 tablespoons Dijon mustard

2 teaspoons dried thyme

½ teaspoon dried rosemary

1 cup plain low-fat Greek yogurt

¼ cup chopped fresh parsley

3 cups cooked brown rice, warmed

PER SERVING (ABOUT 1 CUP BEEF TIPS, ½ CUP BROWN RICE)
Total Calories: 342; Total Fat: 16g; Saturated Fat: 4g; Cholesterol: 43mg; Sodium: 298mg; Potassium: 486mg; Total Carbohydrate: 29g; Fiber: 2g; Sugars: 2g; Protein: 21g

1. In a large skillet over medium-high heat, heat 2 tablespoons of olive oil until it shimmers.

2. Season the meat with salt and pepper. Add it to the skillet and sear on all sides until deeply browned, 3 to 5 minutes per side. Using tongs, remove the meat from the pan and set aside.

3. Return the skillet to the heat and add the remaining 2 tablespoons of olive oil; heat the oil until it shimmers.

4. Add the mushrooms and red onion. Cook for 5 to 7 minutes, stirring occasionally, until deeply browned.

5. Return the meat to the pan. Add the garlic. Cook for 30 seconds, stirring constantly.

6. In a small bowl, whisk the chicken broth, mustard, thyme, and rosemary. Add the sauce to the skillet and stir, scraping up any browned bits from the bottom of the pan. Bring to a simmer and reduce the heat to medium-low. Simmer for 5 minutes, or until the liquid is reduced by half.

7. Stir in the yogurt. Cook, stirring, to heat through. Remove from the heat and stir in the parsley. Serve over the brown rice.

VARIATION TIP: Replace the brown rice with 1 cup zucchini noodles. Use a vegetable peeler to peel long strips from a zucchini. Heat in the microwave for 2 minutes to soften before adding to the sauce at the end.

Spaghetti Squash and Meatballs

SERVES 4   PREP TIME: 10 MINUTES   COOK TIME: 1 HOUR

DIABETES FRIENDLY • GLUTEN FREE • KIDNEY FRIENDLY

This twist on the classic spaghetti and meatballs is a great way to get your veggies. Spaghetti squash has a texture quite similar to spaghetti pasta when cooked as described—you might not even notice your meal is pasta free. If this is a new vegetable to you, do not fear. See the cooking tips for additional ways to prepare it.

1 spaghetti squash, halved lengthwise and seeded

8 ounces 95% extra-lean ground beef

6 garlic cloves, minced

2 tablespoons Italian seasoning

½ teaspoon red pepper flakes

¼ teaspoon sea salt

1 tablespoon extra-virgin olive oil

1 recipe Pesto Sauce (page 154)

PER SERVING (ABOUT ½ CUP SQUASH, ¼ CUP SAUCE, 3 MEATBALLS)
Total Calories: 353; Total Fat: 26g;
Saturated Fat: 5g; Cholesterol: 40mg;
Sodium: 302mg; Potassium: 334mg;
Total Carbohydrate: 17g; Fiber: 4g;
Sugars: 5g; Protein: 17g

1. Preheat the oven to 400°F.
2. Place the squash halves, cut-side down, on a rimmed baking sheet. Bake for 50 to 60 minutes until soft.
3. Turn squash over. Draw a fork across the flesh of the squash to create noodle-like strands. Set aside.
4. While the squash cooks, in a large bowl combine the ground beef, garlic, Italian seasoning, red pepper flakes, and salt. Form the meat mixture into 12 meatballs.

5. In a large skillet over medium-high heat, heat the olive oil until it shimmers.

6. Add the meatballs. Cook on all sides until done, about 10 minutes total.

7. Add the pesto to the hot spaghetti squash. Top with the meatballs.

COOKING TIP: For longer spaghetti strands, halve the squash crosswise, scoop out the seeds, and cut it into rings. This also reduces cooking time to about 30 minutes. You can also cook spaghetti squash in a slow cooker so it's ready when you arrive home from work. Leave the squash whole and prick it all over with a fork. Put it in a slow cooker with ½ cup water. Cover the cooker and set to low heat. Cook for 8 hours. Split the squash after it is cooked, remove the seeds, and use a fork to pull it into spaghetti-like strands.

Flank Steak Chimichurri with Grilled Vegetables

SERVES 4 PREP TIME: 10 MINUTES COOK TIME: 15 MINUTES

DIABETES FRIENDLY • GLUTEN FREE

Chimichurri is a flavorful Argentinian sauce similar to pesto that's often served with beef. If you don't have an outdoor grill, use a grill pan or cook these kebabs in the oven. Roast them in a 350°F oven on a rimmed baking sheet for about 30 minutes, turning every 7 to 10 minutes.

½ **cup fresh Italian parsley**

¼ **cup extra-virgin olive oil**

2 garlic cloves, minced

¼ **teaspoon red pepper flakes**

¼ **teaspoon ground cumin**

¼ **teaspoon kosher salt**

3 tablespoons red wine vinegar

**12 ounces beef flank steak,
    cut into 1-inch cubes**

1 zucchini, cut into thick slices

12 cherry tomatoes

1 red onion, cut into large chunks

1. Preheat a grill to high heat. Soak 12 wooden skewers in water.

2. In a blender or food processor, combine the parsley, olive oil, garlic, red pepper flakes, cumin, salt, and red wine vinegar. Blend until a paste forms. Set aside.

3. Alternating ingredients, thread the beef, zucchini, and tomatoes onto the skewers. Place the skewers on the grill. Cook for about 4 minutes per side until the beef is cooked through.

4. Brush the chimichurri on the meat when it is done cooking. Serve with additional sauce on the side.

PER SERVING (3 KEBABS)
Total Calories: 289; Total Fat: 20g;
Saturated Fat: 4g; Cholesterol: 30mg;
Sodium: 203mg; Potassium: 620mg;
Total Carbohydrate: 8g; Fiber: 2g;
Sugars: 2g; Protein: 19g

VARIATION TIP: Feel free to use other seasonal veggies, such as bell pepper or yellow squash.

Mediterranean Lamb Rib Chops with Roasted Fennel

SERVES 4   PREP TIME: 10 MINUTES   COOK TIME: 30 MINUTES

DIABETES FRIENDLY • GLUTEN FREE • KIDNEY FRIENDLY

Fennel has a delicious flavor with just a hint of licorice. When roasted, it develops deep savory flavors that serve as the perfect complement to Mediterranean-spiced lamb chops. The lamb rib chops are just the perfect serving size (you'll also see them called lamb lollipops)—they are about 3 ounces each.

2 tablespoons dried oregano

1 teaspoon dried rosemary

1 teaspoon dried thyme

1 teaspoon garlic powder

½ teaspoon sea salt, divided

¼ teaspoon freshly ground black pepper

4 lamb rib chops

2 fennel bulbs, cored and cut into large chunks (see cooking tip)

1 red onion, roughly chopped

4 tablespoons extra-virgin olive oil, divided

PER SERVING (1 RIB CHOP, ½ CUP FENNEL)
Total Calories: 362; Total Fat: 24g;
Saturated Fat: 5g; Cholesterol: 75mg;
Sodium: 433mg; Potassium: 540mg;
Total Carbohydrate: 12g; Fiber: 4g;
Sugars: 1g; Protein: 25g

1. Preheat the oven to 425°F.

2. In a small bowl, stir together the oregano, rosemary, thyme, garlic powder, ¼ teaspoon of salt, and the pepper. Rub the spices on the lamb chops and set them aside.

3. In a large bowl, toss the fennel and red onion with 2 tablespoons of olive oil and the remaining ¼ teaspoon of salt. Spread the vegetables in a single layer on a rimmed baking sheet. Roast for about 30 minutes until golden brown, stirring once during cooking. Remove from the oven and set aside.

4. In a large skillet over medium-high heat, heat the remaining 2 tablespoons of olive oil until it shimmers.

5. Add the lamb chops. Cook for 4 to 5 minutes per side until well browned on each side.

COOKING TIP: To prepare fennel, cut off the celery-like stalks and discard. Cut the core out of the bulb at the bottom using a wedge-shaped cut. Chop the fennel as directed.

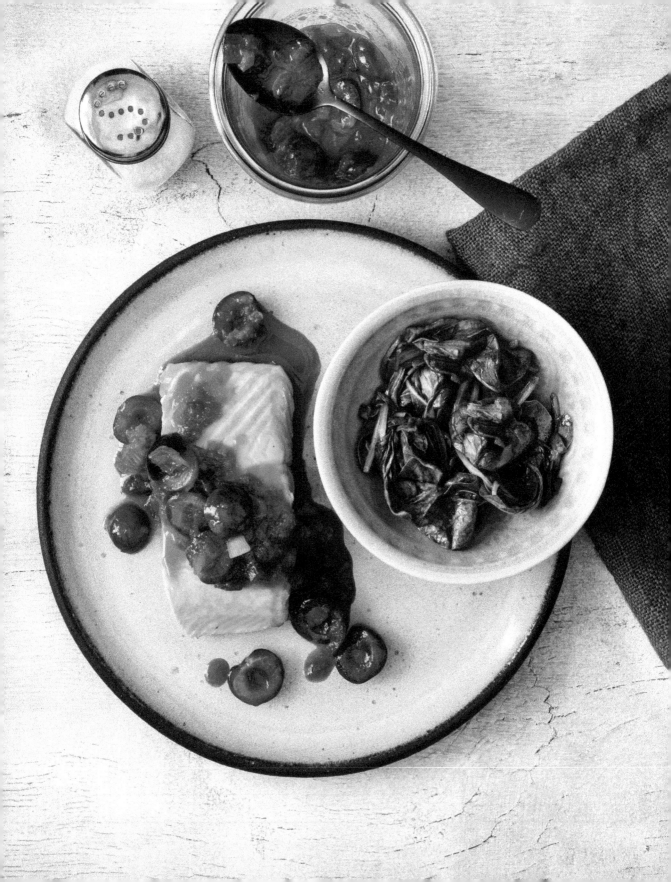

CHAPTER 9

Salmon Cakes with Avocado Salsa

SERVES 4 PREP TIME: 10 MINUTES COOK TIME: 25 MINUTES

DIABETES FRIENDLY

Salmon cakes are delicious with rice and veggies, or they make a great burger. Using fresh salmon is best—let it cool completely before mixing it with the other ingredients. If you use canned salmon, choose low-sodium and rinse it well to remove as much salt as possible before adding it to the cakes.

12 ounces salmon

½ cup finely chopped scallion, white and green parts, divided

2 garlic cloves, minced, divided

2 tablespoons grated peeled fresh ginger, divided

1 large egg, beaten

½ cup whole-wheat bread crumbs

2 tablespoons chopped fresh cilantro

1 tablespoon extra-virgin olive oil

1 avocado, peeled, pitted, and cubed

¼ teaspoon sea salt

Juice of 1 lime

PER SERVING (1 CAKE, ¼ CUP SALSA)
Total Calories: 323; Total Fat: 21g;
Saturated Fat: 3g; Cholesterol: 100mg;
Sodium: 218mg; Potassium: 708mg;
Total Carbohydrate: 14g; Fiber: 5g;
Sugars: 1g; Protein: 22g

1. Preheat the oven to 450°F.

2. Place the salmon, flesh-side down, on a rimmed baking sheet. Bake for about 12 minutes until opaque. Refrigerate to cool. Once cooled, remove the skin and flake the salmon into a bowl.

3. Add ¼ cup of scallion, 1 garlic clove, 1 tablespoon of ginger, the egg, bread crumbs, and cilantro. Gently mix to combine. Form the mixture into 4 patties. Refrigerate for 30 minutes.

4. In a large nonstick skillet over medium-high heat, heat the olive oil until it shimmers, swirling the pan to coat the bottom.

5. Add the salmon cakes. Cook for 3 to 5 minutes per side until browned on both sides.

6. While the salmon cooks, in a small bowl toss the avocado with the remaining ¼ cup of scallion, the remaining garlic clove, the sea salt, and lime juice.

7. Serve the salmon with the avocado spooned over the top.

VARIATION TIP: You can also use 12 ounces of cooked, flaked whitefish here, such as cod.

Shrimp Ceviche

SERVES 4   PREP TIME: 10 MINUTES, PLUS CHILLING TIME

DIABETES FRIENDLY • GLUTEN FREE • KIDNEY FRIENDLY

Shrimp ceviche is a refreshing, light salad with bright citrus flavors and tender baby shrimp. Use precooked baby shrimp and let the ceviche rest in the fridge for an hour or two to allow the flavors to blend. You can adjust the heat by adding more or fewer jalapeños. The white membranes on the inside of the jalapeño are the hottest part of the chili, so remove those and the seeds to make the dish less spicy. It is helpful to wear gloves when cutting chiles to keep the hot oils off your skin.

8 ounces cooked baby shrimp, chilled and rinsed

½ red onion, finely chopped

1 to 2 jalapeño peppers, seeded, ribbed, and finely minced

¼ cup chopped fresh cilantro leaves

1 avocado, peeled, pitted, and cubed

1 cucumber, cubed

24 cherry tomatoes, quartered

Juice of 1 orange

Juice of 1 lime

Juice of 1 lemon

3 garlic cloves, minced or pressed

Pinch cayenne pepper (optional)

1. In a large bowl, combine the shrimp, red onion, jalapeño, cilantro, avocado, cucumber, cherry tomatoes, orange juice, lime juice, lemon juice, garlic, and cayenne (if using). Mix well.

2. Cover and chill for at least 30 minutes, and up to 2 hours.

OPTION: If you have a shellfish allergy or are not partial to shrimp, use 12 ounces of a cooked and cooled flaked whitefish, such as halibut or haddock.

PER SERVING (ABOUT 1 CUP)
Total Calories: 147; Total Fat: 7g; Saturated Fat: 1g;
Cholesterol: 36mg; Sodium: 171mg;
Potassium: 580mg; Total Carbohydrate: 16g;
Fiber: 5g; Sugars: 4g; Protein: 7g

Steamer Clams with Lemon Fennel Broth

SERVES 4   PREP TIME: 10 MINUTES   COOK TIME: 30 MINUTES

DIABETES FRIENDLY • GLUTEN FREE • KIDNEY FRIENDLY

This is really delicious served with a crusty bread to dip into the broth. The broth is fragrant and flavorful, and fennel pairs really well with the clams.

2 tablespoons extra-virgin olive oil

2 tablespoons finely minced shallot

1 fennel bulb and fronds, cored and chopped, separated (see cooking tip)

3 garlic cloves, minced

2½ pounds steamer or Manila clams, rinsed (see ingredient tip)

Juice of 1 lemon

Zest of 1 lemon

3 cups low-sodium chicken broth

PER SERVING (2 CUPS)
Total Calories: 240; Total Fat: 14g; Saturated Fat: 5g; Cholesterol: 50mg; Sodium: 224mg; Potassium: 282mg; Total Carbohydrate: 14g; Fiber: 2g; Sugars: <1g; Protein: 16g

1. In a large pot over medium-high heat, heat the olive oil until it shimmers.
2. Add the shallot and fennel bulb. Cook for about 5 minutes, stirring occasionally, until the fennel begins to soften.
3. Add the garlic. Cook for 30 seconds, stirring constantly.
4. Add the clams, lemon juice and zest, and chicken broth. Cover the pot and cook for 5 to 10 minutes until the clams open. Remove and discard any unopened clams.
5. Stir in the fennel fronds.

INGREDIENT TIP: To rinse the clams, put them in a bowl of water and agitate. Allow the sand to fall to the bottom. Empty the water and add more. Continue this cycle until no sand settles to the bottom of the bowl.

COOKING TIP: The two parts of fennel generally eaten are the white bulb and the wispy green fronds. Cut off the celery-like stalks in between the two and discard them. Cut the core out of the bulb at the bottom using a wedge-shaped cut. For this recipe, chop the bulb and fronds separately as they are added at different times.

Baked Fish and Chips with Tartar Sauce

SERVES 4   PREP TIME: 15 MINUTES   COOK TIME: 30 MINUTES

DIABETES FRIENDLY

Classic fish and chips are high in sodium and fat, especially when you add tartar sauce. This version has an easy, low-fat, homemade tartar sauce and the fish and chips are baked instead of fried. The key to timing here is to cook the potatoes for about 10 minutes before you add the fish, so you can prepare the fish while the potatoes cook.

1 large russet potato, halved lengthwise and cut into ¼-inch-thick wedges

1 tablespoon extra-virgin olive oil

1 tablespoon Mrs. Dash, Original or Lemon Pepper Blend, or any salt-free seasoning you prefer

1 cup whole-wheat bread crumbs

½ cup whole-wheat flour

1 tablespoon dried thyme

1 teaspoon garlic powder

1 teaspoon onion powder

1 teaspoon dried mustard

1 cup low-fat buttermilk

1 large egg, beaten

12 ounces cod, cut into 8 thin pieces

½ cup plain low-fat Greek yogurt

2 tablespoons chopped fresh chives

1 tablespoon finely minced shallot

1 teaspoon dried dill

Zest of 1 lemon

Pinch cayenne pepper

PER SERVING (2 PIECES COD, ¼ POTATO, 2 TABLESPOONS TARTAR SAUCE)
Total Calories: 363; Total Fat: 7g; Saturated Fat: 2g; Cholesterol: 100mg; Sodium: 203mg; Potassium: 449mg; Total Carbohydrate: 43g; Fiber: 5g; Sugars: 5g; Protein: 33g

1. Preheat the oven to 425°F.

2. In a large bowl, toss the potato with the olive oil and Mrs. Dash seasoning. Transfer to a rimmed baking sheet. Bake for about 30 minutes, turning twice during cooking (about every 10 minutes) until crisp on the outside.

3. Meanwhile, in a large zip-top bag, combine the bread crumbs, flour, thyme, garlic powder, onion powder, and dried mustard.

4. In a medium bowl, whisk the buttermilk and egg.

5. Coat the cod in the buttermilk mixture and put it in the zip-top bag. Seal the bag and shake to coat with the bread crumbs. Put the coated cod on a rimmed baking sheet. Bake for about 20 minutes until golden brown.

6. In a small bowl, whisk the yogurt, chives, shallot, dill, lemon zest, and cayenne. Serve the sauce on the side.

VARIATION TIP: This recipe makes delicious chicken nuggets as well. Cut 12 ounces boneless, skinless chicken breast into 8 pieces and follow directions above. Cook for about 30 minutes.

Lemon Pepper Cod with Lemony Sautéed Greens

SERVES 4   PREP TIME: 5 MINUTES   COOK TIME: 15 MINUTES

DIABETES FRIENDLY • GLUTEN FREE • KIDNEY FRIENDLY

It's really easy to make lemon pepper cod. This one-pot version also allows you to cook up a tasty side of greens, and it takes about 20 minutes from start to finish to have a nutritious meal on the table. Feel free to use 12 ounces of any locally available whitefish in place of the cod.

3 tablespoons extra-virgin olive oil, divided

3 cups chopped stemmed kale

Zest of 1 lemon

4 (3-ounce) cod fillets

½ teaspoon freshly ground black pepper

Juice of 2 lemons

PER SERVING (3 OUNCES COD, ½ CUP GREENS)
Total Calories: 201; Total Fat: 11g; Saturated Fat: 1g; Cholesterol: 40mg; Sodium: 93mg; Potassium: 462mg; Total Carbohydrate: 5g; Fiber: 1g; Sugars: <1g; Protein: 21g

1. In a large skillet over medium-high heat, heat 2 tablespoons of olive oil until it shimmers.

2. Add the kale and lemon zest. Cook for about 5 minutes, stirring occasionally, until soft. Remove the kale from the skillet and set aside.

3. Wipe out the skillet with a paper towel and add the remaining 1 tablespoon of olive oil. Return the skillet to medium-high heat and heat the oil until it shimmers, swirling the pan to coat the bottom.

4. Liberally season the cod on both sides with pepper. Carefully add it to the hot oil. Cook for 2 to 3 minutes per side until opaque and cooked through.

5. Squeeze the lemon juice over the top of the fish. Bring to a simmer. Move the cod to the edges of the pan and return the kale to the skillet. Cook for 1 to 2 minutes to heat through.

VARIATION TIP: Lime juice and orange juice are also delicious in this recipe. Use the juice of 3 limes (and the zest of 1) or the juice of 1 orange (and the zest of ½) in place of the lemon juice and zest.

Roasted Halibut with Tropical Black Bean Salsa

SERVES 4   PREP TIME: 10 MINUTES   COOK TIME: 15 MINUTES

DIABETES FRIENDLY • GLUTEN FREE

Halibut has a sweet, mild flavor that's delicious with tropical salsa. Prepare the salsa while the halibut roasts, and you'll have dinner on the table in 15 to 20 minutes. You can refrigerate the salsa and fish for up to 3 days, but store them separately. Reheat the fish in the microwave.

4 (3-ounce) skin-on halibut fillets

1 tablespoon extra-virgin olive oil

¼ teaspoon sea salt

2 cups chopped fresh peaches, or frozen peaches, thawed

½ cup low-sodium canned black beans, drained and rinsed

¼ cup chopped red onion

1 garlic clove, minced

½ jalapeño pepper, seeded and minced

Juice of 1 lime

1 tablespoon chopped fresh cilantro

1. Preheat the oven to 450°F.
2. Place the halibut skin-side down on a rimmed baking sheet. Brush it with the olive oil and sprinkle it with salt. Bake for about 15 minutes until the fish is opaque.
3. While the fish cooks, in a medium bowl, stir together the peaches, black beans, red onion, garlic, jalapeño, lime juice, cilantro, and salt. Mix well. Serve the salsa spooned over the fish.

PER SERVING (3 OUNCES HALIBUT, ¼ CUP SALSA)
Total Calories: 222; Total Fat: 6g; Saturated Fat: 1g; Cholesterol: 35mg; Sodium: 206mg; Potassium: 700mg; Total Carbohydrate: 16g; Fiber: 3g; Sugars: 8g; Protein: 25g

INGREDIENT TIP: If halibut isn't locally available, substitute any whitefish that is, such as haddock or cod.

Almond-Crusted Salmon with Green Beans

SERVES 4   PREP TIME: 10 MINUTES   COOK TIME: 15 MINUTES

DIABETES FRIENDLY • GLUTEN FREE

If you use fresh beans, you'll need to parboil them: Trim off the ends and halve the beans lengthwise. Boil them in water for about 2 minutes. Shock them in a bowl of ice water to stop the cooking and proceed with the recipe. If you use frozen beans, steam them so they are completely thawed before you sauté them.

½ cup almond meal

¼ teaspoon sea salt

Zest of 1 orange

2 tablespoons dried tarragon

4 (3-ounce) salmon fillets

4 tablespoons Dijon mustard

2 tablespoons extra-virgin olive oil

2 tablespoons minced shallot

2 cups fresh or frozen green beans
   (see headnote)

Juice of 1 orange

¼ teaspoon freshly ground black pepper

PER SERVING (3 OUNCES SALMON, ½ CUP GREEN BEANS)
Total Calories: 310; Total Fat: 20g; Saturated Fat: 2g; Cholesterol: 47mg; Sodium: 368mg; Potassium: 676mg; Total Carbohydrate: 12g; Fiber: 3g; Sugars: 5g; Protein: 22g

1. Preheat the oven to 350°F. Line a rimmed baking sheet with parchment paper. Set aside.

2. In a small bowl, stir together the almond meal, salt, orange zest, and tarragon.

3. Place the salmon, skin-side down, on the prepared baking sheet. Spread each piece with 1 tablespoon of mustard and sprinkle evenly with the almond mixture. Bake for about 15 minutes until the salmon is opaque.

4. Meanwhile, in a large skillet over medium-high heat, heat the olive oil until it shimmers.

5. Add the shallot and green beans. Cook for about 5 minutes, stirring frequently, until crisp-tender.

6. Add the orange juice and pepper. Cook for about 5 minutes more until the juice reduces by half.

VARIATION TIP: You can also use 12 ounces of whitefish or trout in place of the salmon.

Salmon with Ginger-Cherry Sauce and Spinach

SERVES 4   PREP TIME: 20 MINUTES   COOK TIME: 40 MINUTES

DIABETES FRIENDLY • GLUTEN FREE

This cherry sauce is a combination of sweet and savory that perfectly complements the flavor of salmon. Make the sauce ahead and let it cool before brushing it on the salmon. It will keep, refrigerated, for up to 5 days, so it's easy to make on the weekend and add it to the salmon midweek to save some time.

4 tablespoons extra-virgin olive oil, divided

2 tablespoons minced shallot

Juice of 2 oranges

Zest of 1 orange

1 tablespoon honey

2 tablespoons grated peeled fresh ginger, divided

¼ teaspoon sea salt

2 cups bing cherries, pitted (see ingredient tip) and quartered

4 (3-ounce) salmon fillets

4 cups fresh spinach

PER SERVING (3 OUNCES SALMON, ¼ CUP COOKED SPINACH)
Total Calories: 343; Total Fat: 20g;
Saturated Fat: 3g; Cholesterol: 47mg;
Sodium: 207mg; Potassium: 889mg;
Total Carbohydrate: 25g; Fiber: 2g;
Sugars: 20g; Protein: 19g

1. In a medium pot over medium-high heat, heat 2 tablespoons of olive oil until it shimmers.

2. Add the shallot. Cook for about 5 minutes, stirring occasionally, until soft.

3. Add the orange juice and zest, the honey, 1 tablespoon of ginger, the salt, and the cherries. Bring to a simmer. Cook for about 10 minutes, stirring occasionally, until the cherries are soft and the liquid is reduced some. Cool completely and divide in half.

4. Preheat the oven to 350°F. Line a rimmed baking sheet with parchment paper.

5. Place the salmon skin-side down on the prepared baking sheet. Brush with half the cherry sauce. Bake for about 15 minutes until opaque.

6. Meanwhile, in a large skillet over medium-high heat, heat the remaining 2 tablespoons of olive oil until it shimmers.

7. Add the spinach and remaining 1 tablespoon of ginger. Cook for 2 to 3 minutes, turning occasionally, until wilted.

8. Reheat the remaining half of the cherry sauce in the microwave or on the stove top. Serve it drizzled over the cooked salmon with the spinach on the side.

VARIATION TIP: If you'd like, use 2 cups broccoli florets instead of the spinach. In a large skillet over medium-high heat, heat the remaining 2 tablespoons of olive oil. Add the broccoli. Sauté for 5 to 7 minutes until browned.

INGREDIENT TIP: To pit cherries quickly, remove the stem, poke a sturdy straw or chopstick tip through the bottom of the cherry, and push the pit out the top.

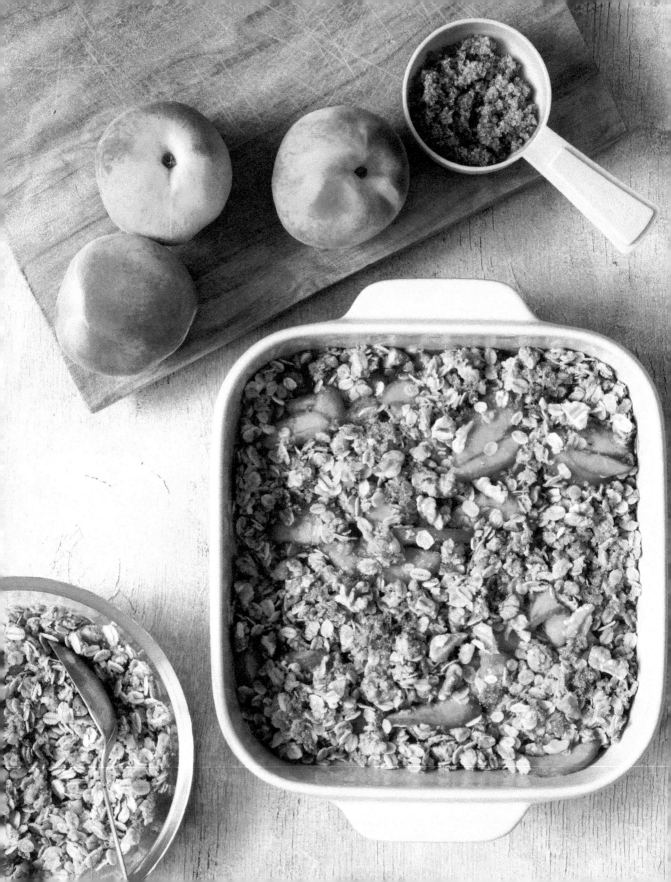

CHAPTER 10

Lemon Curd and Meringue Cups

SERVES 4 PREP TIME: 15 MINUTES, PLUS CHILLING TIME COOK TIME: 15 MINUTES

GLUTEN FREE • KIDNEY FRIENDLY

This is essentially lemon meringue pie without the crust. Baking the meringue separately allows you to store the components separately and assemble just before eating. The meringues can be kept at room temperature in a zip-top bag for up to 5 days. Of course if you'd rather you can simply top the lemon curd with two tablespoons of light whipped cream. You can also substitute any freshly squeezed citrus juice for the lemon, such as orange juice, blood orange juice, or lime juice.

Juice of 2 lemons

½ cup confectioners' sugar

2 large eggs

Zest of 1 lemon

3 large egg whites, at room temperature

¼ teaspoon cream of tartar

Pinch salt

⅓ cup granulated sugar, or 4 packets stevia

PER SERVING (1 RAMEKIN)
Total Calories: 177; Total Fat: 3g;
Saturated Fat: 1g; Cholesterol: 105mg;
Sodium: 115mg; Potassium: 101mg;
Total Carbohydrate: 34g; Fiber: <1g;
Sugars: 32g; Protein: 6g

1. Strain the lemon juice into a small saucepan to remove any pulp. Add the confectioners' sugar. Put the pan over low heat. Cook, stirring, until the sugar dissolves.

2. In a small bowl, using a handheld electric mixer, beat the whole eggs. While beating, pour the lemon and sugar mixture in a thin stream into the bowl. Continue beating for 1 minute once all the mixture is incorporated. Scrape the egg, lemon, and sugar mixture back into the pan and return it to low heat. Add the lemon zest. Cook for 1 to 2 minutes, stirring constantly, until the lemon curd thickens. Pour the mixture into 4 (4-ounce) ramekins. Cover with plastic wrap and chill.

3. Preheat the broiler.

4. In a medium bowl, combine the egg whites, cream of tartar, and salt. Using a handheld electric mixer, beat until they foam. While still beating, 1 tablespoon at a time, add the granulated sugar, or the stevia, 1 packet at a time. Continue beating for 5 to 7 minutes until stiff peaks form. Spoon the meringue, in 4 portions, onto a rimmed baking sheet. Broil for 1 to 3 minutes until browned.

5. Place the meringues onto the chilled lemon curd.

COOKING TIP: You should have about $2/3$ cup lemon juice and 1 teaspoon lemon zest from the lemons.

Chocolate Almond Meringue Cookies

MAKES 18 COOKIES   PREP TIME: 15 MINUTES   COOK TIME: 25 MINUTES

DIABETES FRIENDLY • GLUTEN FREE • KIDNEY FRIENDLY

These cookies are easy to make, but they take a while to bake. The result, however, is light, crisp, chocolatey cookies that are tasty and satisfying. For best results, use an eggbeater or stand mixer to get the right texture on the meringue.

3 large egg whites (see cooking tip)

⅛ teaspoon cream of tartar

Pinch salt

½ teaspoon almond extract

⅔ cup sugar

1 tablespoon unsweetened cocoa powder

PER SERVING (2 COOKIES)
Total Calories: 63; Total Fat: <1g;
Saturated Fat: 0g; Cholesterol: 0mg;
Sodium: 36mg; Potassium: 34mg;
Total Carbohydrate: 15g; Fiber: <1g;
Sugars: 15g; Protein: 1g

1. Preheat the oven to 300°F. Line a baking sheet with parchment paper. Set aside.

2. In a medium bowl, combine the egg whites, cream of tartar, salt, and almond extract. Using a handheld electric mixer, beat until foamy.

3. While still beating, 1 tablespoon at a time, add the sugar. Beat for about 7 minutes until stiff peaks form. Gently fold in the cocoa powder. Spoon the meringue, in 18 portions, onto the prepared baking sheet.

4. Bake for 20 to 25 minutes until the cookies are crisp.

COOKING TIP: When making meringue, fat and temperature can both keep it from reaching stiff peaks. Make sure your bowl and beaters are very clean, and separate the eggs one at a time into separate bowls to make sure you don't wind up with even a dot of yolk in the whites.

Oatmeal and Dried Cranberry Cookies

MAKES 12 COOKIES   PREP TIME: 15 MINUTES   COOK TIME: 10 MINUTES

Cranberries are rich in antioxidants, and oats contain heart-healthy soluble fiber. These oatmeal cookies do include butter, so if you need to watch saturated fat in your diet, pay attention to the serving size noted.

1⅓ cups old-fashioned rolled oats

⅓ cup flaxseed

⅓ cup all-purpose flour

1 teaspoon ground cinnamon

½ teaspoon ground ginger

¼ teaspoon baking soda

¼ teaspoon baking powder

Pinch salt

Zest of 1 orange

6 tablespoons unsalted butter,
    at room temperature

¾ cup packed light brown sugar

1 teaspoon vanilla extract

1 large egg, beaten

¾ cup dried cranberries

PER SERVING (1 COOKIE)
Total Calories: 199; Total Fat: 8g;
Saturated Fat: 4g; Cholesterol: 33mg;
Sodium: 53mg; Potassium: 248mg;
Total Carbohydrate: 35g; Fiber: 3g;
Sugars: 19g; Protein: 3g

1. Preheat the oven to 350°F. Line a baking sheet with parchment paper. Set aside.

2. In a medium bowl, whisk the oats, flaxseed, flour, cinnamon, ginger, baking soda, baking powder, salt, and orange zest. Set aside.

3. In a large bowl, cream together the butter, brown sugar, and vanilla. Stir in the egg.

4. Add the dry ingredients to the wet ingredients, stirring until well combined. Drop by the spoonful into 12 cookies on the prepared baking sheet.

5. Bake for 8 to 10 minutes until the cookies are browned.

MAKE-AHEAD TIP: These freeze well so you can have cookies throughout the week. You can also freeze the dough in single cookies before baking, store them in zip-top bags, and bake one at a time so you can have a warm, fresh cookie to satisfy that sweet tooth.

Honey Lemon Chia Pudding with Blackberries

SERVES 4 PREP TIME: 10 MINUTES, PLUS CHILLING TIME

GLUTEN FREE

Chia seeds, when soaked overnight, thicken and become gelatinous, so they make a really easy and tasty, no-cook pudding. The pudding will keep, refrigerated, for about 4 days, but do not freeze. Sprinkle with fresh blackberries, or berries of your choice, when ready to serve.

6 tablespoons chia seeds

2 cups low-fat milk

2 tablespoons honey

Zest of 1 lemon

1 cup fresh blackberries

PER SERVING (½ CUP)
Total Calories: 191; Total Fat: 6g;
Saturated Fat: <1g; Cholesterol: 7mg;
Sodium: 60mg; Potassium: 166mg;
Total Carbohydrate: 26g; Fiber: 9g;
Sugars: 16g; Protein: 9g

1. In a medium bowl, whisk the chia seeds, milk, honey, and lemon zest. Pour into 4 (4-ounce) ramekins. Cover with plastic wrap and refrigerate overnight.

2. Serve with ¼ cup of blackberries spooned over each pudding.

COOKING TIP: Adjust the thickness of this pudding by adding more liquid (thinner) or more chia seeds (thicker). About 30 minutes before serving, check the pudding to see how the texture is. If it is too thin, add 1 teaspoon of chia seeds and let sit for 30 minutes more. If it's too thick, stir in 1 teaspoon of milk at a time until you reach the desired consistency.

Baked Apple

SERVES 4 PREP TIME: 10 MINUTES COOK TIME: 30 MINUTES

GLUTEN FREE

Baked apples taste best in fall when they are in season. Choose a sweet-tart apple, such as a Honeycrisp, Pink Lady, Cripps Pink, or Braeburn, for the best flavor and texture. Serve with a scoop of low-fat frozen vanilla yogurt or mix 1 tablespoon pure maple syrup and ¼ cup plain low-fat Greek yogurt and spoon over the top of the warm apples if you wish.

4 apples, tops, stem, and core removed (see preparation tip)

¼ cup packed light brown sugar

½ teaspoon ground ginger

½ teaspoon ground cinnamon

4 teaspoons unsalted butter

4 tablespoons chopped walnuts

PER SERVING (1 APPLE EACH)
Total Calories: 226; Total Fat: 9g;
Saturated Fat: 3g; Cholesterol: 9mg;
Sodium: 8mg; Potassium: 283mg;
Total Carbohydrate: 45g; Fiber: 5g;
Sugars: 32g; Protein: 2g

1. Preheat the oven to 350°F.
2. Place the apples, cut-side up, in a small baking dish.
3. In a small bowl, stir together the brown sugar, ginger, and cinnamon. Spoon the mixture into the center of each apple.
4. Top the brown sugar mixture with 1 teaspoon of butter per apple. Sprinkle with the walnuts.
5. Bake for about 30 minutes until the apples are tender.

PREPARATION TIP: To prepare the apples, slice off the top (about ¼ inch) from each apple. Using a spoon or knife, cut out the core, leaving the bottom intact so it forms a "bowl."

Frozen Yogurt with Cherry Compote

SERVES 4 PREP TIME: 10 MINUTES COOK TIME: 10 MINUTES

DIABETES FRIENDLY • GLUTEN FREE

Warm cherry-ginger compote spooned over frozen yogurt makes a delicious dessert, and it's quick and easy to make. Store the compote separately from the yogurt. It doesn't need to be warm to be delicious if you need to make it ahead. It will keep, refrigerated, for up to 5 days.

½ cup freshly squeezed orange juice

1 cup sweet red cherries (such as bing cherries), pitted and quartered (see ingredient tip, page 133)

2 tablespoons sugar

1 teaspoon ground ginger

½ teaspoon ground cinnamon

2 teaspoons cornstarch

2 tablespoons water

4 (¼-cup) scoops low-fat frozen vanilla yogurt

1. In a medium pot over medium-high heat, combine the orange juice, cherries, sugar, ginger, and cinnamon. Cook for about 7 minutes, stirring occasionally, until the cherries are saucy.

2. In a small bowl, whisk the cornstarch and water until smooth. Add this slurry to the simmering sauce. Cook for about 3 minutes more until it begins to thicken.

3. Cool slightly or serve chilled, scooped over the frozen yogurt.

PER SERVING (¼ CUP FROZEN YOGURT, ¼ CUP COMPOTE)
Total Calories: 122; Total Fat: 1g;
Saturated Fat: <1g; Cholesterol: 12mg;
Sodium: 40mg; Potassium: 227mg;
Total Carbohydrate: 25g; Fiber: 1g;
Sugars: 21g; Protein: 5g

VARIATION TIP: If you like, mix the compote, after it is chilled, into ½ cup plain low-fat Greek yogurt.

Brown Sugar Peaches with Oat Walnut Crumble

SERVES 8   PREP TIME: 10 MINUTES   COOK TIME: 30 MINUTES

This warm crumble is fragrant and delicious—it's the ultimate comfort food. You can also substitute nectarines, if you wish, with similar results. Choose a light-tasting oil, such as a light olive oil—don't use extra-virgin, which has too strong of an olive flavor.

8 peaches, peeled, pitted, and sliced (see cooking tip) or frozen peaches, thawed

½ cup packed light brown sugar, divided

1 teaspoon ground ginger

1 teaspoon ground cinnamon

1 cup old-fashioned rolled oats

¾ cup whole-wheat flour

¼ cup chopped walnuts

⅓ cup light olive oil, or canola oil

PER SERVING (¼ CUP)
Total Calories: 274; Total Fat: 13g; Saturated Fat: 1g; Cholesterol: 0mg; Sodium: 6mg; Potassium: 262mg; Total Carbohydrate: 45g; Fiber: 5g; Sugars: 22g; Protein: 4g

1. Preheat the oven to 350°F.
2. In a large bowl, gently stir together the peaches, ¼ cup of brown sugar, the ginger, and cinnamon. Transfer to a 9-inch-square baking pan or deep-dish pie pan.
3. In a small bowl, stir together the oats, flour, walnuts, remaining ¼ cup of brown sugar, and olive oil. Sprinkle the mixture over the top of the peach mixture.
4. Bake for about 30 minutes until the peaches bubble and the topping is browned. Serve warm or chilled.

COOKING TIP: To peel peaches easily, put the peaches in a pot of boiling water for 10 to 20 seconds, or until the skin splits. Plunge them into ice water to stop the cooking. The peels will slip off easily with a paring knife.

Panna Cotta with Blueberries

SERVES 4   PREP TIME: 10 MINUTES, PLUS CHILLING TIME   COOK TIME: 6 MINUTES

DIABETES FRIENDLY • GLUTEN FREE • KIDNEY FRIENDLY

Panna cotta is like a creamy gelatin. It's lightly sweet once it sets up, and it makes a delicious treat. While it's quick and easy to make, you'll need to chill for about 8 hours so the panna cotta can set. You can make the blueberry sauce ahead and refrigerate it as well.

¼ cup cold water

2½ teaspoons unflavored gelatin (or
   1 envelope Knox unflavored gelatin)

2 cups low-fat milk

½ teaspoon almond extract

Zest of 1 orange

4 tablespoons sugar, divided

Juice of 1 orange

1 cup fresh or frozen blueberries

¼ teaspoon cornstarch

PER SERVING (¼ CUP)
Total Calories: 66; Total Fat: <1g;
Saturated Fat: <1g; Cholesterol: 4mg;
Sodium: 33mg; Potassium: 31mg;
Total Carbohydrate: 12g; Fiber: <1g;
Sugars: 11g; Protein: 3g

1. Put the cold water in a small saucepan and sprinkle the gelatin over the top. Let sit for about 3 minutes. Stir. Put the pan over medium heat. Cook for 1 to 2 minutes, stirring, until the gelatin thoroughly dissolves.

2. Add the milk, almond extract, orange zest, and 3 tablespoons of sugar. Cook for about 3 minutes, stirring, until the sugar dissolves. Pour the mixture into 4 (4-ounce) ramekins. Cover with plastic wrap and refrigerate overnight until the panna cotta sets.

3. In a small saucepan over medium heat, combine the orange juice, blueberries, remaining 1 tablespoon of sugar, and cornstarch. Bring to a simmer, stirring constantly. Cook for about 5 minutes until the blueberries are soft and the sauce is thickened. Chill.

4. Spoon the blueberry sauce over the panna cotta to serve.

VARIATION TIP: If you don't like the flavor of almonds, omit the almond extract and use vanilla in its place. Omit the orange zest too. This will make a vanilla panna cotta with blueberry sauce.

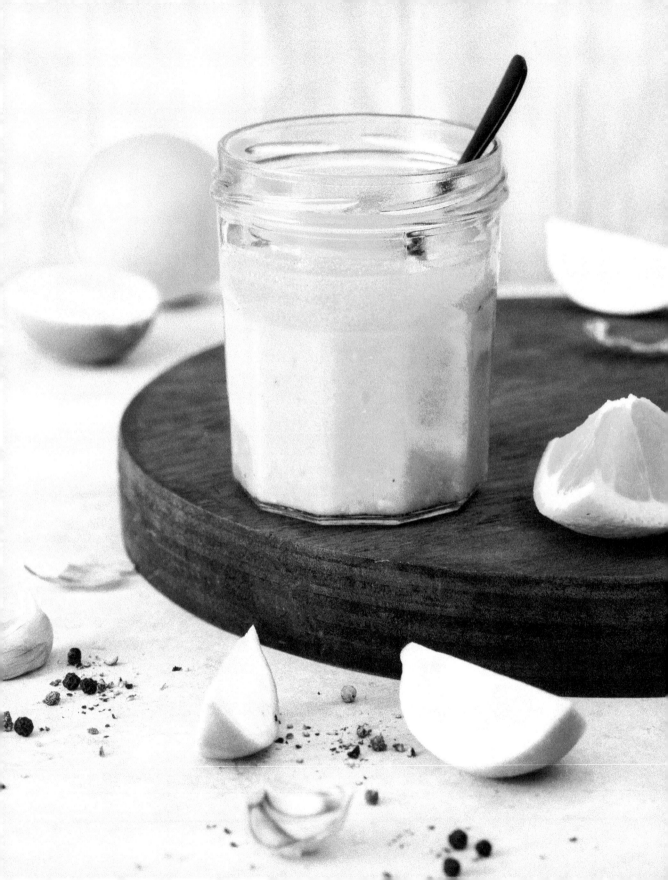

CHAPTER 11

Poultry Broth

MAKES 6 CUPS   **PREP TIME: 15 MINUTES**   **COOK TIME: 12 TO 24 HOURS**

DIABETES FRIENDLY • GLUTEN FREE • KIDNEY FRIENDLY

Use this unsalted chicken broth in any recipes that call for low-sodium chicken broth. Freeze in 1-cup serving portions for up to 12 months and thaw on the stove top as needed. It also makes a great base for soups and sauces.

2 pounds chicken or turkey wings, backs, or necks

2 carrots, peeled and chopped

2 celery stalks, chopped

1 onion, quartered

6 garlic cloves, smashed

8 peppercorns

1 teaspoon dried thyme

7 cups water

PER SERVING (1 CUP)
Total Calories: 24; Total Fat: <1g;
Saturated Fat: 0g; Cholesterol: 0mg;
Sodium: 34mg; Potassium: 169mg;
Total Carbohydrate: 5g; Fiber: 1g;
Sugars: 2g; Protein: 1g

1. In a slow cooker, combine the chicken parts, carrots, celery, onion, garlic, peppercorns, thyme, and water. Cover the cooker and set to low heat. Cook for 12 to 24 hours. The longer it cooks, the more flavor and nutrients are extracted from the ingredients.

2. Strain and discard the solids. Cover the broth and refrigerate it overnight.

3. In the morning, skim the fat from the top of the broth. Discard the fat. Refrigerate in an airtight container for up to 5 days.

INGREDIENT TIP: You can also use a chicken carcass from a roasted chicken or turkey to make this broth.

Citrus Vinaigrette

MAKES ½ CUP   PREP TIME: 5 MINUTES

DIABETES FRIENDLY • GLUTEN FREE • KIDNEY FRIENDLY • VEGAN

This dressing is delicious on salads, dark leafy greens, and steamed veggies. It makes a flavorful marinade for fish as well. To boost flavor, add a tablespoon of chopped fresh herbs, such as thyme, rosemary, or tarragon.

2 tablespoons freshly squeezed lemon juice

2 tablespoons freshly squeezed orange juice

2 tablespoons freshly squeezed lime juice

2 tablespoons extra-virgin olive oil

1 teaspoon Dijon mustard

1 garlic clove, minced

¼ teaspoon sea salt

⅛ teaspoon freshly ground black pepper

In a small bowl, combine the lemon, orange, and lime juices, olive oil, mustard, garlic, salt, and pepper. Whisk until smooth. Refrigerate in an airtight container for up to 5 days.

PREPARATION TIP: The mustard acts as an emulsifier to hold the fat and citrus juice together. Use this trick in any vinaigrette you make to hold it together better.

PER SERVING (2 TABLESPOONS)
Total Calories: 73; Total Fat: 7g; Saturated Fat: 1g;
Cholesterol: 0mg; Sodium: 177mg;
Potassium: 85mg; Total Carbohydrate: <1g;
Fiber: 0g; Sugars: 1g; Protein: 0g

Asian Vinaigrette

MAKES ½ CUP   PREP TIME: 5 MINUTES

DIABETES FRIENDLY • KIDNEY FRIENDLY • VEGAN

Because this recipe includes Chinese hot mustard, it is not gluten free (Chinese mustard contains wheat flour). For a slightly less spicy, gluten-free version, replace the Chinese mustard with Dijon mustard. Use this on salads, slaws, or as a meat or poultry marinade or toss it with steamed veggies for some extra flavor.

¼ cup apple cider vinegar

2 tablespoons freshly squeezed lime juice

½ teaspoon sriracha, or to taste (optional)

½ teaspoon Chinese hot mustard

2 tablespoons extra-virgin olive oil

1 garlic clove, minced

2 tablespoons chopped, fresh cilantro

1 tablespoon grated peeled fresh ginger

¼ teaspoon sea salt

In a small bowl, combine the vinegar, lime juice, sriracha (if using), mustard, olive oil, garlic, cilantro, ginger, and salt. Whisk until smooth. Refrigerate in an airtight container for up to 1 week.

PREPARATION TIP: Omit the sriracha if you don't prefer spice. If you like lots of spice, add up to ½ teaspoon more, which will add 40 mg of sodium.

PER SERVING (2 TABLESPOONS)
Total Calories: 71; Total Fat: 7g; Saturated Fat: 1g;
Cholesterol: 0mg; Sodium: 151mg;
Potassium: 40mg; Total Carbohydrate: 1g;
Fiber: <1g; Sugars: <1g; Protein: <1g

Blackberry Vinaigrette

MAKES ½ CUP   PREP TIME: 5 MINUTES

DIABETES FRIENDLY • GLUTEN FREE • KIDNEY FRIENDLY • VEGAN

Sweet and savory, this vinaigrette is especially delicious on bitter or peppery greens, such as frisée or arugula. It's also delicious used as a fish marinade. To make a tasty fish or poultry sauce, briefly simmer it with ½ teaspoon of cornstarch.

½ cup fresh blackberries (do not use frozen)

2 tablespoons apple cider vinegar

2 tablespoons extra-virgin olive oil

1 garlic clove, minced

1 tablespoon minced shallot

¼ teaspoon sea salt

⅛ teaspoon freshly ground black pepper

PER SERVING (2 TABLESPOONS)
Total Calories: 72; Total Fat: 7g; Saturated Fat: 1g; Cholesterol: 0mg; Sodium: 146mg; Potassium: 52mg; Total Carbohydrate: 3g; Fiber: 1g; Sugars: 1g; Protein: <1g

In a blender or food processor, combine the blackberries, vinegar, olive oil, garlic, shallot, salt, and pepper. Blend until smooth. Refrigerate in an airtight container for up to 3 days.

VARIATION TIP: Add up to 1 tablespoon chopped fresh herbs, such as rosemary or thyme, to change the flavor. You can also spice it up by adding up to ½ teaspoon red pepper flakes, a pinch at a time, to get the heat to your liking.

Greek Yogurt Southwestern Dressing

MAKES ABOUT ¾ CUP   PREP TIME: 5 MINUTES

DIABETES FRIENDLY • GLUTEN FREE • KIDNEY FRIENDLY • VEGETARIAN

One delicious dressing, so many choices—top a taco or taco salad, serve with greens, dip fresh veggies, or jazz up a burrito.

½ cup plain low-fat Greek yogurt

Juice of 1 lime

Pinch cayenne pepper

1 teaspoon chili powder

1 small tomato, finely chopped

½ teaspoon ground coriander

In a blender or food processor, combine the yogurt, lime juice, cayenne, chili powder, tomato, and coriander. Blend until smooth. Refrigerate in an airtight container for up to 5 days (do not freeze).

VARIATION TIP: Jazz this dressing up with chopped scallion, 1 minced garlic clove, or 2 tablespoons chopped, fresh cilantro.

PER SERVING (ABOUT 3 TABLESPOONS)
Total Calories: 32; Total Fat: <1g; Saturated Fat: <1g; Cholesterol: 4mg; Sodium: 21mg; Potassium: 95mg; Total Carbohydrate: 3g; Fiber: <1g; Sugars: 1g; Protein: 3g

Ginger Stir-Fry Sauce

MAKES ½ CUP   PREP TIME: 5 MINUTES

DIABETES FRIENDLY • KIDNEY FRIENDLY • VEGAN

When preparing this, be sure to use low-sodium soy sauce; if you're gluten intolerant, use low-sodium gluten-free soy sauce (regular soy sauce contains wheat). Add this sauce to any stir-fry or use with veggies, meat, or seafood.

2 tablespoons grated peeled fresh ginger (see ingredient tip)

1 tablespoon low-sodium soy sauce

Juice of 1 lime

3 garlic cloves, minced

½ teaspoon sesame oil

¼ teaspoon chili oil

½ teaspoon cornstarch

In a small bowl, combine the ginger, soy sauce, lime juice, garlic, sesame oil, chili oil, and cornstarch. Whisk until smooth. Refrigerate in an airtight container for up to 1 week. Before using, whisk to reincorporate the cornstarch.

INGREDIENT TIP: To grate fresh ginger, peel it with a vegetable peeler and use a rasp-style grater.

PER SERVING (2 TABLESPOONS)
Total Calories: 21; Total Fat: 1g; Saturated Fat: <1g; Cholesterol: 0mg; Sodium: 145mg; Potassium: 41mg; Total Carbohydrate: 2g; Fiber: <1g; Sugars: <1g; Protein: <1g

Pesto Sauce

MAKES ABOUT ¾ CUP   PREP TIME: 5 MINUTES

DIABETES FRIENDLY • GLUTEN FREE • KIDNEY FRIENDLY • VEGETARIAN

Serve this zippy sauce on pasta or to top fish, meat, or poultry. You can change the herbs and use the same basic portions to create variations. For example, make a lemon arugula pesto by using ¼ cup arugula and the zest of 1 lemon.

¼ cup fresh basil leaves

¼ cup grated Parmesan cheese

3 tablespoons extra-virgin olive oil

Pinch red pepper flakes

2 garlic cloves, minced

¼ cup walnuts

PER SERVING (ABOUT 3 TABLESPOONS)
Total Calories: 162; Total Fat: 17g;
Saturated Fat: 3g; Cholesterol: 5mg;
Sodium: 85mg; Potassium: 51mg;
Total Carbohydrate: 2g; Fiber: 1g;
Sugars: 0g; Protein: 3g

In a food processor, combine the basil, Parmesan, olive oil, red pepper flakes, garlic, and walnuts. Process until smooth. Keep refrigerated in an airtight container. This is best eaten the first day or two after making.

VARIATION TIP: Replace the walnuts with pecans, pine nuts, or almonds. The flavor will change slightly, but it's still delicious.

Basic Marinara Sauce

MAKES ABOUT 1 CUP   PREP TIME: 10 MINUTES   COOK TIME: 15 MINUTES

DIABETES FRIENDLY • GLUTEN FREE • VEGAN

Marinara is a basic, fresh-tasting tomato sauce. It's delicious on whole-wheat pasta and is good with any type of meat. This low-sodium version is easy and quick to make.

2 tablespoons extra-virgin olive oil

1 shallot, minced, or about ¼ cup minced red onion

6 garlic cloves, minced (see ingredient tip)

1 (15.5-ounce) can no-salt-added crushed tomatoes, undrained

1 tablespoon dried Italian seasoning

⅛ teaspoon red pepper flakes

¼ teaspoon sea salt

¼ cup chopped fresh basil, or fresh Italian parsley

PER SERVING (ABOUT ½ CUP)
Total Calories: 190; Total Fat: 14g;
Saturated Fat: 2g; Cholesterol: 0mg;
Sodium: 318mg; Potassium: 660mg;
Total Carbohydrate: 16g; Fiber: 4g;
Sugars: 6g; Protein: 4g

1. In a medium pot over medium-high heat, heat the olive oil until it shimmers.
2. Add the shallot. Cook for about 5 minutes, stirring occasionally, until soft.
3. Add the garlic. Cook for 30 seconds, stirring constantly.
4. Stir in the tomatoes, Italian seasoning, red pepper flakes, and salt. Bring to a simmer. Cook for 7 minutes, stirring occasionally.
5. Stir in the basil.
6. Refrigerate leftovers in an airtight container for up to 5 days, or freeze for up to 6 months.

INGREDIENT TIP: One of the easiest ways to peel and mince a lot of garlic is to put the unpeeled pieces, one at a time, into a garlic press and press them into a bowl. Remove the peels from the press between garlic cloves.

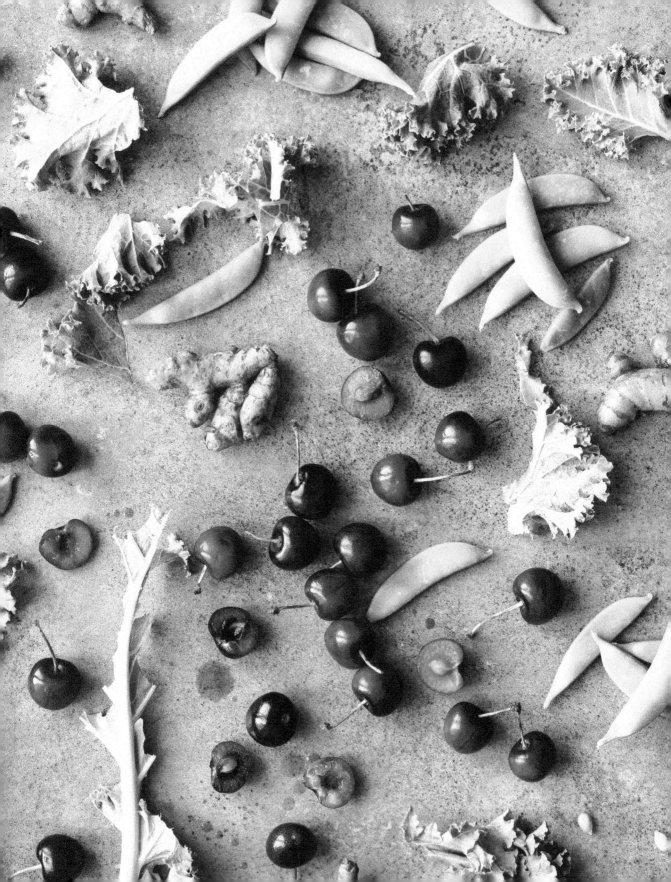

MEASUREMENT CONVERSIONS

VOLUME EQUIVALENTS (LIQUID)

US STANDARD	US STANDARD (OUNCES)	METRIC (APPROXIMATE)
2 tablespoons	1 fl. oz.	30 mL
¼ cup	2 fl. oz.	60 mL
½ cup	4 fl. oz.	120 mL
1 cup	8 fl. oz.	240 mL
1½ cups	12 fl. oz.	355 mL
2 cups or 1 pint	16 fl. oz.	475 mL
4 cups or 1 quart	32 fl. oz.	1 L
1 gallon	128 fl. oz.	4 L

OVEN TEMPERATURES

FAHRENHEIT	CELSIUS (APPROXIMATE)
250°F	120°C
300°F	150°C
325°F	165°C
350°F	180°C
375°F	190°C
400°F	200°C
425°F	220°C
450°F	230°C

VOLUME EQUIVALENTS (DRY)

US STANDARD	METRIC (APPROXIMATE)
⅛ teaspoon	0.5 mL
¼ teaspoon	1 mL
½ teaspoon	2 mL
¾ teaspoon	4 mL
1 teaspoon	5 mL
1 tablespoon	15 mL
¼ cup	59 mL
⅓ cup	79 mL
½ cup	118 mL
⅔ cup	156 mL
¾ cup	177 mL
1 cup	235 mL
2 cups or 1 pint	475 mL
3 cups	700 mL
4 cups or 1 quart	1 L

WEIGHT EQUIVALENTS

US STANDARD	METRIC (APPROXIMATE)
½ ounce	15 g
1 ounce	30 g
2 ounces	60 g
4 ounces	115 g
8 ounces	225 g
12 ounces	340 g
16 ounces or 1 pound	455 g

REFERENCES

Abhishek, A., M. Doherty. "Education and Non-Pharmacological Approaches for Gout." *Rheumatology* 57, no. Suppl. 1 (January 1, 2018): i51–i58. doi:10.1093 /rheumatology/kex421.

Bardin, T., P. Richette. "Impact of Comorbidities on Gout and Hyperuricemia: An Update on Prevalence and Treatment Options." *BMC Medicine* 15, no. 123 (July 2017). doi:10.1186/s12916-017-0890-9.

Bove, M., A. Cicero, M. Veronesi, et al. "An Evidence-Based Review on Urate-Lowering Treatments: Implications for Optimal Treatment of Chronic Hyperuricemia." *Vascular Health and Risk Management* 2017, no. 13 (February 2017): 23–28. doi.org/10.2147 /VHRM.S115080.

Burns, C. M., R. L. Wortmann. "Latest Evidence on Gout Management: What the Clinician Needs to Know." *Therapeutic Advances in Chronic Disease* 3, no. 6 (November 2012): 271–286. doi:10.1177/2040622312462056.

Chandrate, P., C. Mallen, E. Roddy, et al. "You Want to Get on with the Rest of Your Life: A Qualitative Study of Health-Related Quality of Life in Gout." *Clinical Rheumatology* 35 (2016): 1197–1205. doi:10.1007/s10067-015-3039-2.

Choi, H. K., D. B. Mount, A. M. Reginato, et al. "Pathogenesis of Gout." *Annals of Internal Medicine* 143, no. 7 (October 2005): 499–516.

Choi, H. K., G. Curham. "Soft Drinks, Fructose Consumption, and the Risk of Gout in Men: Prospective Cohort Study." *BMJ* 336, no. 7639 (February 7, 2008): 309–312. doi:https://doi.org/10.1136/bmj.39449.819271.BE.

Choi, H. K., K. Atkinson, E. Karlson, et al. "Purine-Rich Foods, Dairy, and Protein Intake, and the Risk of Gout in Men." *New England Journal of Medicine* 350, no. 11 (March 11, 2004): 1093–103.

Choi, H. K., K. Atkinson, E. W. Karlson, et al. "Alcohol Intake and Risk of Incident Gout in Men: A Prospective Study." *Lancet* 363, no. 9417 (April 2004): 1277–1281.

Choi, H. K., W. Willett, and G. Curhan. "Fructose-Rich Beverages and the Risk of Gout in Women." *Journal of the American Medical Association* 304, no. 20 (November 24, 2010): 2270–2278. doi:10.1001/jama.2010.1638.

Dowell, A., C. Morris, L. Macdonald, et al. "I Can't Bend It and It Hurts like Mad: Direct Observation of Gout Consultations in Routine Primary Health Care." *BioMed Central Family Practice* 18 (October 2017): 91. doi:10.1186/s12875-017-0662-9.

García-Pérez, L. E., M. Alvarez, T. Dilla, et al. "Adherence to Therapies in Patients with Type 2 Diabetes." *Diabetes Therapy: Research, Treatment, and Education of Diabetes and Related Disorders* 4, no. 2 (December 2013): 175–94. doi:10.1007 /s13300-013-0034-y.

Hamburger, M., H. S. Baraf, T. C. Adamson, et al. "2011 Recommendations for the Diagnosis and Management of Gout and Hyperuricemia." *The Physician and Sportsmedicine* 39, no. 4 (November 2011): 98–123. doi:10.3810/psm.2011.11.1946.

Harris, MD, L. B. Siegel, and J. A. Alloway. "Gout and Hyperuricemia." *American Family Physician* 59, no. 4 (February 15, 1999): 925–34.

Harrold, L. R., K. M. Mazor, D. Peterson, et al. "Patients' Knowledge and Beliefs Concerning Gout and Its Treatment: A Population-Based Study." *BioMed Central Musculoskeletal Disorders* 13 (2012): 180. doi:10.1186/1471-2474-13-180.

Juraschek, S. P., A. C. Gelber, H. K. Choi, et al. "Effects of the Dietary Approaches to Stop Hypertension (DASH) Diet and Sodium Intake on Serum Uric Acid." *Arthritis and Rheumatology* 68, no. 12 (December 2016): 3002–3009. doi:10.1002/art.39813.

Kanbara, A., M. Hakoda, and I. Seyama. "Urine Alkalization Facilitates Uric Acid Excretion." *Nutrition Journal* 9, no. 45 (2010). https://doi.org/10.1186/1475-2891-9-45.

Kelley, D., Y. Adkins, and K. D. Laugero. "A Review of the Health Benefits of Cherries." *Nutrients* 10, no. 3 (March 2018): 368. https://doi.org/10.3390/nu10030368.

Khanna, D., J. D. FitzGerald, P. P. Khanna, et al. "2012 American College of Rheumatology Guidelines for Management of Gout Part I: Systematic Non-Pharmacologic and Pharmacologic Therapeutic Approaches to Hyperuricemia." *Arthritis Care and Research* 64, no. 10 (October 2012): 1431–1446. doi:10.1002/acr.21772.

Khanna, D., P. P. Khanna, J. D. FitzGerald, et al. "2012 American College of Rheumatology Guidelines for Management of Gout Part 2: Therapy and Anti-Inflammatory Prophylaxis of Acute Gouty Arthritis." *Arthritis Care and Research* 64, no. 10 (October 2012): 1447–1461. doi:10.1002/acr.21773.

Kim, S. C., J. Liu, and D. H. Solomon. "Risk of Incident Diabetes in Patients with Gout: A Cohort Study." *Arthritis and Rheumatology* 67, no. 1 (January 2015): 273–280. doi:10.1002/art.38918.

Krishnan, E., D. Lienesch, and C. K. Kwoh. "Gout in Ambulatory Care Settings in the United States." *Journal of Rheumatology* 35, no. 3 (March 2008): 498–501.

Kuehn, Bridget M. "Chronic Disease Approaches Needed to Curb Gout's Growing Burden." *Journal of the American Medical Association* 319, no. 13 (April 3, 2018): 1307–1309. doi:10.1001/jama.2018.0547.

Mandell, B. F. "Clinical Manifestations of Hyperuricemia and Gout." *Cleveland Clinic Journal of Medicine* 75, Supplement 5 (July 2008): S5–8.

National Kidney Foundation. "A Clinical Update on Gout: Optimizing Care for Patients with Chronic Kidney Disease." www.kidney.org/sites/default/files/02-10-6446_ABE_Gout_Bulletin_SINGLE_PAGES.pdf.

National Kidney Foundation: "Gout and Hyperuricemia in Chronic Kidney Disease: What Is Clinically Significant?" www.kidney.org/sites/default/files/02-10-6972_JBF_Hyperurecemia_Bulletin_singlepg.pdf.

Neogi, T., T. Jansen, N. Dalbeth, et al. "2015 Gout Classification Criteria: An American College of Rheumatology/European League Against Rheumatism Collaborative

Initiative." *Arthritis and Rheumatology* 67, no. 10 (October 2015): 2557–2568. doi:10.1002/art.39254.

Nielsen, S., E. Bartels, M. Henriksen, et al. "Weight Loss for Overweight and Obese Individuals with Gout: A Systematic Review of Longitudinal Studies." *Annals of the Rheumatic Diseases* 76, no. 11 (November 2017): 1870–1882. doi:10.1136 /annrheumdis-2017-211472.

Nuki, G. "An Appraisal of the 2012 American College of Rheumatology Guidelines for the Management of Gout." *Current Opinion in Rheumatology* 26, no. 2 (March 2014): 152–61. doi:10.1097/BOR.0000000000000034.

Perez-Ruiz, F., and G. Desideri. "Improving Adherence to Gout Therapy: An Expert Review." *Therapeutics and Clinical Risk Management* 14 (May 2018): 793–802. https://doi.org/10.2147/TCRM.S162956.

Ragab, G., M. Elshahaly, and T. Bardin. "Gout: An Old Disease in New Perspective— A Review." *Journal of Advanced Research* 8, no. 5 (September 2017): 495–511. doi:10.1016/j.jare.2017.04.008.

Rai, S. K., T. T. Fung, N. Lu, et al. "The Dietary Approaches to Stop Hypertension (DASH) Diet, Western Diet, and Risk of Gout in Men: Prospective Cohort Study." *BMJ* (Clinical Research Edition) 357 (May 9, 2017): j1794. doi:10.1136/bmj.j1794.

Rho, Y. H., Y. Zhu, and H. K. Choi. "The Epidemiology of Uric Acid and Fructose." *Seminars in Nephrology* 31, no. 5 (September 2011): 410–419. doi:10.1016 /j.semnephrol.2011.08.004.

Roddy, E., and H. K. Choi, "Epidemiology of Gout." *Rheumatic Diseases Clinics of North America* 40, no. 2 (May 2014): 155–175. doi:10.1016/j.rdc.2014.01.001.

Ruilope, L., and C. Cerezo. "Uric Acid and Cardiovascular Risk Considered: An Update." An article from the e-journal of the European Society of Cardiology, *Cardiology Practice* 10, no. 21 (March 2012).

Rymal, E., and D. Rizzolo. "Gout: A Comprehensive Review." *Journal of the American Academy of Physician Assistants* 27, no. 9 (September 2014): 26–31. doi:10.1097 /01.JAA.0000453233.24754.ec.

Sacks, F. M., L. P. Svetkey, W. M. Vollmer, et al. "Effects on Blood Pressure of Reduced Dietary Sodium and the Dietary Approaches to Stop Hypertension (DASH) diet. DASH-Sodium Collaborative Research Group." *New England Journal of Medicine* 344, no. 1 (January 2001): 3–10.

Schlesinger, N., M. A. Detry, B. K. Holland, et al. "Local Ice Therapy During Bouts of Acute Gouty Arthritis." *Journal of Rheumatology* 29, no. 2 (February 2002): 331–4.

Schlesinger, N., "Response to Application of Ice May Help Differentiate Between Gouty Arthritis and Other Inflammatory Arthritides." *Journal of Rheumatology* (December 2006): 275-6.

Schumacher, H. R. "Patient Education: How Can We Improve It and Evaluate the Effects?" *Journal of Clinical Rheumatology* 17, no. 5 (August 2011): 229–230 doi:10.1097/RHU.0b013e31822d9a51.

Seoyoung, K. C., J. Liu, and D. H. Solomon. "Risk of Incident Diabetes in Patients with Gout: A Cohort Study." *Arthritis and Rheumatology* 67, no. 1 (January 2015): 273–280. doi:10.1002/art.38918.

Shekelle, P. G., J. FitzGerald, S. J. Newberry, et al. "Management of Gout." *Comparative Effectiveness Reviews No. 176* (March 2016). Agency for Healthcare Research and Quality (Rockville, MD, U.S.) NCBI Bookshelf. A service of the National Library of Medicine, National Institutes of Health. www.ncbi.nlm.nih.gov/books/NBK356145 /#results.s30.

Singh, J. "Gout and Comorbidity: A Nominal Group Study of People with Gout." *Arthritis Research and Therapy* 19 (September 15, 2017): 204. doi:10.1186 /s13075-017-1416-8.

Skerrett, P. J., and W. C. Willett. "Essentials of Healthy Eating: A Guide." *Journal of Midwifery and Women's Health* 55, no. 6 (November–December 2010): 492–501. doi:10.1016/j.jmwh.2010.06.019.

Tang, O., E. R. Miller, A. C. Gelber, et al. "DASH Diet and Change in Serum Uric Acid over Time." *Clinical Rheumatology* 36, no. 6 (June 2017): 1413–1417. doi:10.1007/s10067-017-3613-x.

Taylor, E. N., M. J. Stampfer, D. B. Mount, et al. "DASH-Style Diet and 24-Hour Urine Composition." *Clinical Journal of American Society of Nephrology* 5, no. 12 (December 2010): 2315–2322. doi:10.2215/CJN.04420510.

Teng, G. G., A. Pan, J. M. Yuan, and W. P. Koh. "Food Sources of Protein and Risk of Incident Gout in the Singapore Chinese Health Study." *Arthritis and Rheumatology* 67, no. 7 (July 2015): 1933–42. doi:10.1002/art.39115.

Whelton, P. K., R. M. Carey, W. S. Aronow, et al. "2017 ACC/AHA/AAPA/ABC/ACPM/AGS/APhA/ASH /ASPC/NMA/PCNA Guideline for the Prevention, Detection, Evaluation, and Management of High Blood Pressure in Adults: A Report of the American College of Cardiology/American Heart Association Task Force on Clinical Practice Guidelines." *Journal of the American College of Cardiology* 71, no. 19 (May 2018): 2199–2269. doi:10.1016/j.jacc.2017.11.005.

Zhang, Y., C. Chen, H. K. Choi, et al. "Purine-Rich Foods Intake and Recurrent Gout Attacks." *Annals of the Rheumatic Diseases* 71, no. 9 (2012):1448–53.

Zhang, Y., T. Neogi, C. Chen, et al. "Cherry Consumption and Decreased Risk of Recurrent Gout Attacks." *Arthritis and Rheumatism* 64, no. 12 (December 2012): 4004–11. doi:10.1002/art.34677.

Zhu, Y., B. J. Pandy, and H. K. Choi. "Prevalence of Gout and Hyperuricemia in the U.S. General Population: The National Health and Nutrition Examination Survey 2007–2008." *Arthritis and Rheumatism* 63, no. 10 (October 2011):3136–3141. doi:10.1002/art.30520.

UPTODATE.COM (SUBSCRIPTION REQUIRED)

Becker, Michael A., MD. "Asymptomatic Hyperuricemia." UpToDate.com. Accessed 8/23/18. www.uptodate.com/contents/asymptomatic-hyperuricemia?csi =0c8a7950-c856-4f04-b341-d28d325dbcfd&source=contentShare.

Becker, Michael A., MD. "Clinical Manifestations and Diagnosis of Gout." UpToDate. com. Accessed 8/23/18. www.uptodate.com/contents/clinical-manifestations -and-diagnosis-of-gout?csi=514e9f3c-b393-475c-962e-77c3c0153b09&source =contentShare.

Becker, Michael A., MD. "Gout (Beyond the Basics)." UpToDate.com. Accessed 8/26/18. www.uptodate.com/contents/gout-beyond-the-basics?csi=de3e6f15-9224-4cd4-be9d -550f26bfb51d&source=contentShare.

Becker, Michael A., MD. "Lifestyle Modification and Other Strategies to Reduce the Risk of Gout Flares and Progression of Gout." UpToDate.com. Accessed 8/2/18. www.uptodate.com/contents/lifestyle-modification-and-other-strategies-to-reduce -the-risk-of-gout-flares-and-progression-of-gout?csi=15cdc18f-2dfe-43b3-9c65 -55f49c070ca9&source=contentShare.

Becker, Michael A., MD. "Pathophysiology of Gout." UpToDate.com. Accessed 8/23/18. www.uptodate.com/contents/pathophysiology-of-gout?csi=f21c33d3-716c-4ce5-97a3 -3087752f0ce9&source=contentShare.

Becker, Michael A., MD. "Pharmacologic Urate Lowering Therapy and Treatment of Tophi in Patients with Gout?" UpToDate.com. Accessed 8/23/18. www.uptodate .com/contents/pharmacologic-urate-lowering-therapy-and-treatment-of-tophi -in-patients-with-gout?csi=ef314531-ae72-4f49-9ab6-c82f2856c7fc&source =contentShare.

Becker, Michael A., MD. "Treatment of Gout Flares." UpToDate.com. Accessed 8/22/18. www.uptodate.com/contents/treatment-of-gout-flares?csi=501bf27a-6680-430d-a18e-6645eacc8e91&source=contentShare.

Becker, Michael A., MD."Urate Balance." UpToDate.com. Accessed 8/23/18. www.uptodate.com/contents/urate-balance?csi=5f49dffa-d8d5-4892-8548-d105ab7b4410&source=contentShare.

RESOURCES

APP

National Kidney Foundation, Gout Central: Kidney.org/apps/patients /gout-central

WEBSITES

Academy of Nutrition and Dietetics: EatRight.org

American College of Rheumatology: Rheumatology.org

Anti-Inflammatory Diet: DrWeil.com/diet-nutrition/anti-inflammatory-diet -pyramid/dr-weils-anti-inflammatory-food-pyramid

Arthritis Foundation: Arthritis.org

DASH Diet: NHLBI.NIH.gov/health-topics/dash-eating-plan

MedlinePlus. "Vitamin C." MedlinePlus.gov/ency/article/002404.htm

National Institutes of Health: LiverTox.NIH.gov/Colchicine.htm

National Kidney Foundation: Kidney.org/atoz/content/gout/patient-facts

United States Food and Drug Administration: FDA.gov

USDA National Nutrient Database: NDB.NAL.USDA.gov/ndb

WebMd: WebMd.com

RECIPE INDEX

INDEX

ACKNOWLEDGMENTS

I would like to thank Callisto Media for extending the opportunity to fulfill my personal aspiration to write a book. Profound thanks to the entire Callisto team with a special shout out to Vanessa Putt for finding me! My deepest praise and thanks to my editor, Salwa Jabado, for calmly mentoring me through unchartered waters with great patience and an endless stream of support and guidance.

With sincere appreciation, I would also like to acknowledge two exceptional dietitians—Kate Scarlata, RDN, and Melissa Herrmann Dierks, RDN. Their generous nature and ongoing support have afforded me professional growth opportunities for which I am most grateful. They are esteemed colleagues as well as cherished friends.

And lastly, my heartfelt expression of love and deep gratitude for my other half, David Walko. His essence is filled with boundless generosity, kindheartedness, dependability, integrity, and selflessness that lights my way. He's the analytical, practical Virgo who balances my creative, unconventional Aquarian spirit. While we may defy astrological compatibility tables, we grow together as we learn from one another, each and every day.

ABOUT THE AUTHOR

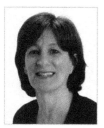 **Sophia Kamveris, MS, RD, LDN,** is a Boston-based registered dietitian and licensed nutritionist with a diverse, 35-year career in the health care field. Having held a series of clinical and management positions with Marriott International, she ultimately found her passion for teaching while working with the U.S. Air Force. As an integrated medical team member, she prescribed dietary and lifestyle recommendations for military personnel to ensure their optimal health was achieved and performance directives were met.

Today, Sophia maintains a private practice and provides individualized nutrition consultations. She specializes in diabetes, cardiovascular disease, and obesity/weight management, and also administers counsel on women's health, digestive disorders, and general health and wellness interests.

Sophia can be reached on her website at EatRightBoston.com.